Catheters, Slurs, and Pickup Lines

Catheters, Slurs, and Pickup Lines

Professional Intimacy in Hospital Nursing

Lisa C. Ruchti

TEMPLE UNIVERSITY PRESS
PHILADELPHIA

TEMPLE UNIVERSITY PRESS
Philadelphia, Pennsylvania 19122
www.temple.edu/tempress

Library of Congress Cataloging-in-Publication Data

Ruchti, Lisa C. (Lisa Camille), 1970–
    Catheters, slurs, and pickup lines : professional intimacy in hospital nursing / Lisa C. Ruchti.
    p. cm.
    Includes bibliographical references and index.
    ISBN 978-1-4399-0752-8 (hardback : alk. paper) — ISBN 978-1-4399-0753-5 (paper : alk.
paper) — ISBN 978-1-4399-0754-2 (e-book)   1. Nurse and patient.   2. Nursing—Social
aspects.   I. Title.
    RT86.3.R83 2012
    610.73—dc23

                                                                                          2011042477

∞ The paper used in this publication meets the requirements of the American National Standard for
Information Sciences—Permanence of Paper for Printed Library Materials, ANSI Z39.48-1992

Printed in the United States of America

2 4 6 8 9 7 5 3 1

To Patrick and Simon

Contents

Acknowledgments

I have never been a nurse or worked in a medical setting. As a result, I could not have written this book without the guidance, interest, and intellectual support of the many nurses I had the pleasure to stand by, follow, and share a cup of coffee with. Their continued enthusiasm for my research sustained me throughout this study. I honor their experiences in, insight about, and commitment to the very difficult and worthy labor of professionally intimate care. I thank the hospital staff and administration for their interest in and support of this study. I am grateful for their investment in their nurses and in hospital care. I appreciate the time and knowledge that, in spite of their busy schedules, all the hospital directors and executives willingly shared with me. Their openness significantly contributed to my methodological and conceptual progress throughout my fieldwork.

I thank the staff at Temple University Press, especially my editor, Mick Gusinde-Duffy. I appreciate his steadfast vision, his commitment to this project, and the ease with which we have worked together. I thank my students at West Chester University, especially Rachel Gottlieb, Rebecca Richman, and Sherrie Ruppersberger, who helped me analyze the data from my interviews with the hospital administrators. Working as part of this research team during my second semester is one of my fondest memories of this project and of my career to date. I also earnestly thank my friends and colleagues in the Women's and Gender Studies Program at West Chester, especially Jen Bacon, Joy Fritschle, Karin Gedge, Erin Hurt, Lisa Kirschenbaum, Rodney Mader, Adale

Sholock, Chris Stangl, Linda Stevenson, and Hyoejin Yoon. I am equally grateful to my friends and colleagues in the Department of Anthropology and Sociology at West Chester, especially Helen Berger, Patti Hite, Susan Johnston, Douglas McConatha, Paul Stoller, and Jackie Zalewski. In administration, I especially thank Mike Ehi Awewoh, Darla Spence Coffey, Jackie Hodes, Becky Mason, Pat Phillips, Barb Schneller, Pam Sheridan, Catherine Spaur, and Lori Vermeulen. Each of these individuals provided me intellectual inspiration, motivation, time, levity, and support throughout this project.

I thank Kathleen Blee, my dissertation advisor in the Sociology Department at the University of Pittsburgh, for her unwavering guidance and astute mentorship. I also thank my committee members, Cecilia Green, Akiko Hashimoto, and Ellen Olshansky, for their individual and collective wisdom. I am also indebted to the faculty of the Women's Studies Program, especially Kathryn Flannery and Lisa Parker, and my wonderful community of friends at the University of Pittsburgh. First and foremost, I thank Melissa Swauger for being my confidant, ally, brilliant consultant, and soul sister. Along with the rest of our crew—Maria Jose Alvarez, Ashley Currier, Kathleen Bulger Gray, Margee Kerr, Connie Oxford, and Dana Reinke—she offered me friendship and guidance that carried me through graduate school and other milestones in my life. An Andrew W. Mellon Pre-dissertation Fellowship, a University of Pittsburgh Provost Fellowship, the University of Pittsburgh Women's Studies Program, the West Chester University College of Arts and Sciences, the West Chester University Department of Anthropology and Sociology, and the West Chester University Women's and Gender Studies Program provided financial support for this research.

I thank my family—my parents, Rick and Peggy Straight, for being my first teachers; my sister, Stacy Cone; my nieces, Alexis and Dannae; my grandmother, Adele Ludek; and the entire Ruchti tribe—for their continued support, encouragement, and patience with what my niece Alexis dubbed my "homework." I am grateful that, although we live far apart, I am, in my heart, always close to home.

Last and most ardently, I thank and commend my beautiful son, Patrick, and my coparent, best friend, and esteemed colleague, Simon Ruchti. I (personally) and this research (generally) benefited immeasurably from Simon's consistent insight and steadfast commitment to seeing this project through and from Patrick's drum playing, dancing, and merrymaking. I take full responsibility for the content of this book, which I earnestly and passionately dedicate to them.

Introduction

Fantasies and Realities in Nursing Care

Anna,[1] a new Latina nurse, prepared for what was next on her shift: she had to go change a catheter for Alan, a young white man. As she gathered her materials, Anna thought about how uncomfortable she had felt the first time she changed a catheter as a nursing student. She marveled about how it did not bother her anymore, but it did sometimes still make her nervous. "When did that change?" she wondered. Anna considered the various ways she could act with her patient during the procedure. When she first asked her mentor, Jason, about this, he suggested she could try not talking as a symbolic way of showing her respect for her patient's privacy. However, Anna knew that talking could serve to help keep her patient's mind on something else. From talks with senior nurses, she was beginning to understand that establishing some intimate connection with her patients was necessary for them to feel safe and to feel better, and it seemed to help patients trust her and the hospital. She did not want to seem "uncaring" like her colleague, Joyce, another new nurse, who avoided intimacy with her patients whenever possible. At the same time, she admitted she did not quite understand how to be professional and intimate at the same time. What if Alan does something she is not prepared for? What if he becomes aroused? What if he feels violated? What if he does not like Chicanas? Should she involve Maura, his wife? Would that make him more or less comfortable with the situation?

Inserting Alan's catheter went well. As she performed the procedure, Anna asked Alan personal questions and shared some information about herself. They discovered that they were both army brats as children and could relate to each other on this personal level. Alan seemed fine when she was finished. He breathed a sigh of relief and thanked Anna. She asked if there was anything else she could do. Maura said, "Um, no Anna, we think you are great. We were just wondering when we would see Alan's nurse—you know, the one in charge of his care. We have some questions about his diagnosis, his procedures, and when he might see the doctor." Anna half-smiled and said a little hesitantly, "I am your nurse" and pointed to her badge. Both Alan and Maura appeared embarrassed. Alan looked away, and Maura blushed. At the same time that Maura started apologizing for their mistake, Anna said, "I can get you another nurse if that would make you more comfortable." "Oh no, that isn't necessary," Maura said. "We just didn't realize . . ." she trailed off. Anna was embarrassed and worried, but she put those feelings aside and reasserted professionalism. She offered to sign Maura up for the hospital's patient advocacy program, PAL. She explained Alan's plan for the day. She promised to tell them both when they could expect Alan's physician.

Although Anna knew she had handled herself well, she left the room feeling frazzled. Did she do something to make Alan and Maura think she was not their nurse? Perhaps she should have brought in her clipboard? Maybe she should wear her name tag in a more prominent place? Then again, she knew she had introduced herself to them that morning as their nurse. Her name was on the board in their room, indicating she was the RN. How could they not know?

Anna was assigned Alan the next day, and unfortunately, things took a turn for the worse. Alan's illness had progressed, and he was feeling significant pain. When Anna went to check on him, she found a very worried-looking Maura and a very frustrated Alan. Alan cried out that he needed his medication. Anna gently explained that he was not due for his medication for another two hours. Alan was furious. He told her that she was so nice yesterday; he just thought she would care for him when he needed it. He started yelling at Anna, cursing at her, using racist and sexist slurs, and saying derogatory things like "Why don't you go back to where you came from?" Anna was shocked. Feelings of humiliation and anger poured over her. When she left the room, Alan called out, asking for a "real" nurse. Anna was especially embarrassed because Alan's room was right next to the nurses' station. Anna could not help but notice that several staff members heard Alan, including her charge nurse Lydia. She worried about how Alan's behavior would reflect on how Lydia would perceive her abilities and professionalism.

After she calmed down, Anna thought about what to do. Although she was taught patients would act out and perhaps call her names, in nursing school Anna was not trained on how to handle such situations. She knew that Alan's anger was coming from a place of pain, but she did not think she could tolerate his accusations, especially the racial slurs and the sexist remarks. Yet she worried that if she told her charge nurse, she would seem unprofessional or unable to handle her job. She knew that other nurses watched her to see what she could handle as a new nurse. She thought that rather than go to her charge nurse, she could say something to Alan herself. She could ask him to stop, but she did not want to upset him or Maura. They were already suffering. Besides, she was not sure he would stop just because she asked him to. He was the patient, after all. He was essentially paying for her services. She decided to ignore Alan's behavior and hoped he would stop.

To Anna's relief, Lydia approached her that evening to ask her what had happened. Although the hospital did not have a formal, transparent approach to addressing prejudicial treatment from patients and similar conflicts, Lydia had a reputation for not tolerating poor treatment of her nurses. Anna was thankful that Lydia was the charge nurse working that night. First, Lydia suggested that if Alan used racist or sexist slurs against her again, she confront the behavior. Anna was nervous about doing this, but Lydia coached her through it and promised she would support her. Lydia insisted this kind of interaction would not make Anna look bad. Anna agreed to try. The next time Alan called her names, she told him to stop. She did not yell at Alan. She just looked him directly in the eye and said, "Alan, the way you talk to me is inappropriate. I am your nurse. Don't do it again." Alan looked angry, but he did not behave angrily. Instead, he rolled his eyes and said, "You're too pretty to be mean to anyway. Maybe you can make it up to me in another way." Anna cringed at the sexual innuendo as Alan winked at her. She looked away and avoided the gaze of Maura, who was sitting there the entire time.

The Fantasy of Care: Naturalizing Intimate Care in the Profession of Nursing

When I first began designing this study while living in Pittsburgh, Pennsylvania, I took a picture of a bus advertisement that read, "Born to be a nurse" (see Appendix C). In it, a little girl of color uses a stethoscope to listen to her teddy bear's heart. This advertisement and others like it suggest that nursing is a natural aspiration for a little girl. It is also noteworthy that the little girl in the advertisement is one of color. It could symbolize the legislative and industry efforts to diversify nursing along racial and ethnic lines. In spite of these efforts and a long-standing nursing shortage in the United States, extremely low numbers of women of color persist in the ranks.[2]

Historians and sociologists explain race stratification in nursing by showing how racism in nursing education and professional associations reduced structural opportunities for women of color, especially in the twentieth century.[3] Over time, white women became and remained the public face of nursing, ideologically and structurally, while women of color occupied primarily low-wage, backroom care work jobs, responsible for the "dirty" work.[4] Sociologists explain this stratification by focusing on how dominant ideologies about women of color shape their material circumstances in professional care work.[5] Moreover, the United States has a long history of recruiting immigrant women of color to work in the United States without addressing discrimination, hate rhetoric, or violence.[6] Rather than address systematic discrimination, recruitment programs emphasize how nursing is a good job for women because women are naturally caring.

There is a long history in nursing that suggests people define good nurses by how much they appear to be naturally good at caring. This lineage in nursing parallels the logic that suggests women are inherently caring.[7] The belief that women are natural caregivers is partially rooted in how women have traditionally provided the bulk of care work in and outside the home. Nurses, administrators, and educators in my study also participated in this naturalizing rhetoric. I found, and my study participants agreed, that patients defined their nursing experience by focusing on care and using words like *nice* and *compassionate* to describe their nurses.[8] Similarly, nurses and hospital administrators mostly talked about "being caring" as a value, rather than as professional work. I suggest that a dichotomy of professionalism and care persists in part because intimacy, as a part of bedside care, seems unprofessional.[9] Indeed, most nurse directors in my study hesitated to use the word *intimacy* to describe their labor. In fact, when I used the word with administrators to ask about work conditions, they grimaced and redirected the conversation to professional care. I was not surprised to learn that the function of intimacy and how it creates and sustains quality health care is virtually invisible in nursing education and in public discussions about practice.[10]

Everyone in my study valued good care, but when asked to explain it, each person had trouble. Nurses and administrators reduced the meaning and circumstances of care work to "being caring." This inability to articulate the process of intimate care work helps maintain what I call the fantasy of care. In the fantasy of care, good care involves almost no conflict between the nurse and patient. When conflict occurs, nurses are naturally adept at handling it in ways that consistently make the patient feel safe. At the same time, it is hard to imagine conflict because the fantasy suggests that caregivers are naturally adept at caring, and care receivers are eternally grateful for the care they receive. For the patient, the fantasy is that care will always be pleasant, welcoming, and warm. The fantasy of care for the nurse is that the care the nurse provides will be both natural and professional. The fantasy of care locates care in the social imagination as a universal experience that can be recognized only when individuals experience it. It serves as a principal value for nursing care but does not reflect the patterns of professional practice. In my study, this fantasy was shared by patients, family members, nurses, and hospital administrators. It naturalized, glorified, and ultimately erased intimate caring behaviors and care work.

The fantasy of care suggests that care always feels good. The reality of care, however, includes how nurses negotiate trust and conflict so that patients trust them. While care may feel natural to the patient, it is actually a series of intimate acts that nurses purposefully and professionally perform to construct this feeling of naturalness. As exemplified by the experience of Anna described at the beginning of this Introduction, in some cases patients act out in abusive and exploitative ways during the provision of emotionally and physically intimate care. The analysis in this book shows how patients, as they become more familiar with their nurses, sometimes cross professional boundaries in an attempt to get their needs met. The principle that care always feels good is well meaning, but as a practice it proves unrealistic. Ignoring how this principle fails also denies the experiences of nurses and limits the analysis of meanings of professional care.

Conflict is not a new idea in nursing.[11] What is new in this book is how I theorize conflict as part of the provision of intimate care. I highlight intimacy in the provision of professional care, which reveals how nurses negotiate conflict with patients. I watched bedside nurses define conflict from patients as inherent to illness or injury and as something that good nurses could overcome. These explanations of conflict were talked about as if common knowledge. I most often heard these explanations when I watched nurses collectively strategize conflict resolution as a team or unit. Much of professional nursing, however, consists of individual practices with patients. When I interviewed nurses, each thought his or her individual experience of intimate conflict with patients was a unique experience that could not be shared with peer nurses and administrators. When I asked why, many shrugged and indicated in some way that it did not occur to them to disclose this information to anyone or that they did not have the time to discuss it. Other nurses told me they worried that talking negatively about patients would make them appear like bad nurses who could not handle the stress of the job. These responses made sense to me. In the first case, individual nurses considered patient conflict a part of the job and believed there was nothing to be done about it except to endure it during care work. In the second case, individual nurses resisted talking about conflict because each thought handling conflict independently was a sign of professionalism.

Catheters, Slurs, and Pickup Lines: Negotiating Mundane, Insulting, and Sexualized Intimacies

Before Anna entered Alan's room, she strategized on how she would make intimate care *seem* natural to Alan and not like professional work that required training. A catheterization was one of the many mundane, intimate procedures Anna would perform on patients. These procedures did not feel intimate to her; any discomfort she may have felt was in part lessened by her focus on providing medical care. She had learned in school how to consider care from her patient's perspective and the importance of combining compassion with skill while performing catherizations, IVs, baths, and other nursing acts that involve physical touch. Anna anticipated that Alan might feel nervous about the intimate nature of this procedure because it involved touch that is personally intimate in any other situation. At the same time, she was not sure how to be professional and intimate simultaneously. She was unsure of what outcome to expect because she was not certain how Alan would react to her. She discussed with Jason and other senior nurses how to make patients like Alan feel comfortable during the process of intimate care.[12] For the catheterization to be successful, Alan needed Anna to be at ease with providing intimate care or, in other words, to seem naturally good at it.

In my research, I discovered that "good" nurses were actually experienced nurses who over time had learned to create a sense of familiarity with their patients as a strategy for gaining trust. I refer to such strategies as *intimate trust*. Although she was a new nurse, Anna had modeled her behavior after experienced nurses. She successfully garnered a sense of familiarity with Alan by sharing some personal information about herself and asking questions of him. Partly because of this success, the catheterization went flawlessly. What might have appeared like a natural ability to care was actually a conscious, strategic use of intimate trust in a professional manner. In other words, Anna employed intimate trust so she could effectively execute her professional labor.

I found that nurses helped patients through their fear of hospitals, doctors, illnesses, and health-care systems to accomplish trust. This trust was necessary so patients could receive quality health care. If patients did not trust their care providers, they would resist procedures, policies, and practices that would help them recover. Once trust was gained, it could be lost at any time. Experienced nurses used intimate trust to work through conflicts that arose from patients' mistrust, feelings of entitlement, and inflated sense of familiarity with nurses. They skillfully negotiated a return to trust so that patients could receive optimal health care.

On the second day Anna was assigned to Alan, after his illness had progressed, Anna experienced her patient angrily yelling racist slurs, making sexist remarks, and using a crude pickup line that could have resulted in a slap to the face in any other context. These acts are forms of *intimate conflict* because they represent a specific kind of intimate labor that nurses encounter as they work to sustain trust with their patients. I learned that an additional form of conflict occurred when patients mistook their nurse's role. For example, when patients misunderstood the position of women of color nurses, new nurses like Anna internalized these misunderstandings and wondered what they could have done to cause them in the first place. Some nurses must first establish and defend their status as nurses for intimate care work to even begin. Alan and Maura thought that Anna was not their nurse. As a result, Anna had to negotiate her feelings about this interaction and simultaneously do more work to professionally gain Alan and Maura's trust. I explain other such instances in this book. I also describe cases where patients outright refused women of color nurses. In each of these cases, nurses were forced to tolerate this treatment, compartmentalize it, and strategize on how to continue care and reestablish intimate trust.

Whether conflict came from patients' fear, anger, entitlement, or increased familiarity with their nurses, I observed a significant pattern in the ways it was a part of intimate labor. Anna did not know how to handle this treatment. She told me she was never taught how to handle these kinds of conflicts with patients. Anna felt threatened, fearful, and frustrated, combined with a concern that Alan would not receive her care. She worried that this disconnect with Alan was her fault and would make her look like a bad nurse who could not care for patients. She did not know how to navigate the racism and sexism that affected her individual practice.

Although much of nursing is valued as an individualized profession, some of the best practices I observed were when the nurses worked together as a team. As Anna considered her next step, Lydia approached her. This simple act relieved Anna from multiple contradictory pressures. Anna did not have to focus on whether her superiors would judge her harshly. Instead, Lydia created a culture that advocated respect for nurses and showed Anna how to care for patients within that context. Lydia offered Anna immediate guidance on how to handle the conflict at hand and simultaneously demonstrated that negotiating intimate care in nursing can be a collective practice, rather than something that nurses must handle alone. While new nurses felt unprepared to handle intimacy or conflict, I observed, experienced nurses handled such situations with professional ease. Over time, I watched senior nurses take new nurses under their wings and *teach* them how to care. Although these experienced nurses insisted that caring could not be taught, they demonstrated otherwise. Without acknowledgment (from themselves or others), they modeled how to handle intimacy and conflict with patients. They negotiated with the harassing patient, the demanding family member, and the intimate moment. I watched how, in contrast to the idea that nurses eat their young, experienced nurses nurtured new nurses by teaching them how to professionally negotiate intimate care for patients.

The primary goal of this book is to mark the professionally intimate labor of nurses that is invisible, naturalized, and taken for granted yet contributes greatly to quality health care and to hospital profit. Although the administrators in my study used traditional definitions of care to describe intimacy in nursing (in part, to avoid using the word *intimacy*), I learned that senior nurses strategically and skillfully negotiated intimacy as part of care work. In school, nurses learned technical skills, therapeutic communication, and care theory; however, school did not entirely prepare them for how patients would not necessarily recognize these skills. I observed new nurses become rudely awakened to the realities of intimate care work once they got on the floor. They did not fully understand the degree to which care included intimate and uncomfortable situations and the extent to which patients would express and exhibit fear and pain through disrespect, demands, and abuse. I found that new nurses were not prepared to handle intimate conflict with patients in part because learning how to manage conflict that is inherent to care contradicts the fantasy of care.[13]

The Study

Anna's story is one example of many in this book that demonstrate how the provision of professionally intimate care in nursing is both invisible and socially constructed.[14] She was one of forty-five nurses whom I interviewed and observed over an eight-month period to study the relationship between intimacy and professional care.[15] I also interviewed ten administrators and three nursing professors on the meanings of intimacy in nursing and whether they thought "being caring" could be taught in nursing school. I designed this study to consider the influence of intersections of race, gender, nationality, and sexuality in part to reflect the increasing diversity in nursing but also because work and other everyday life experiences are constructed by these social factors.[16]

I conducted eight hundred hours of ethnographic observations in a hospital with a diverse nursing staff in a large, growing city in the southwestern region of the United States, close to the Mexico border. This choice offered me a midsize hospital and a nursing staff diverse in race, age, gender, and nationality. I selected the hospital in part because it was a Magnet hospital. The Magnet designation of the American Nurses Association (ANA) is a prestigious award given to approximately 2 percent of hospitals in the United States. It was established in part because the ANA sought to understand and reward hospitals that excelled at recruiting and retaining nurses. It indicates to patients that they will receive quality nursing care and assures nurses of a work environment that values and respects them and provides resources for giving the best care to patients. That I conducted my research in a hospital ranked in the top 2 percent for nursing in the United States helps position my model of professional intimacy as one that is exemplary of skilled and professional intimate nursing care. I chose the city because it is one of the fastest growing cities in the country and is located in a state that faces one of the worst nursing shortages in the country. As such, the state actively sought to recruit minority and male nurses.

At the time of my study, the city had clear divisions—and tensions—along lines of nationality, race, and class (and these divisions remain). The city is in a border state with a significant proportion of native Spanish speakers. The state's Latino and Latina population grew from 19 percent of the total population in 1990 to more than 33 percent in 2003. At the time of the study, the state was home to twenty-two Native American tribes. Real estate and financial planning were booming industries that served affluent individuals who moved there to retire, but there was also a significant homeless population.

To capture how social dynamics shaped by gender, race, and nationality affect individuals' experiences, I use feminist standpoint theory. Feminist standpoint theory argues that people who are closest to everyday interactions, but possess less structural power than those in dominant groups, should contribute to theory about those interactions. In other words, as researchers, we should seek meaning about social life through a "bottom-up" analytical lens as well as a "top-down" analytical lens.[17] I centrally consider the knowledge of bedside nurses because I believe the perspectives of those closest to the experience of providing intimate care can offer knowledge about meanings of care that other observers cannot see. Therefore, I developed the ideas in this book with and on behalf of nurses, from their experiences and as they understood their experiences.

Most of the nurses I interviewed, observed, and informally talked with were bedside nurses and as such had a unique perspective on patient care. These nurses represent the "frontline" nurses; they assess patients, coordinate and explain care plans to patients and their families, and are the first people to manage changes in care for patients. This means that when there is a change in the patient's health, the bedside nurse is the first to know. I believe the experiences of bedside nurses can help all people interested in quality health care understand the nuances of providing intimate care. These nuances include how bedside nurses individually and collectively negotiate conflict with their patients.

Professional Intimacy

The analysis in this book and the model of professional intimacy that results capture how experienced nurses build and sustain trust with their patients. Although it is not recognized, nurses construct intimacy as part of managing care. When managing care, nurses do more than coordinate technical and medical information related to a patient's condition. Much of this management incorporates physical and emotional intimacy, which nurses must also manage to keep their patients' trust. Nurses must have sound medical knowledge and skills, but trust also defines what quality health care is and is not. I mark professional intimacy in organizational processes of care work because naming the process of intimate care will help make visible the skill and experience required when one "gives care" in a professional work setting. I hope that naming this labor will help improve nurse recruitment and retention. Identifying professional intimacy will increase the social and economic value of care, which nurses have identified as crucial to quality health care. I suggest that rather than being born to care, people learn how to care over time and in different contexts.

The phrase *professional intimacy* is peppered throughout the published literature in the fields of business and the therapeutic sciences to indicate how professionals mix professionalism with personal engagement and simultaneously make appropriate boundaries. The goal in this literature is to distinguish between professional and personal relationships, but none of it explicitly describes how to do this. For example, a nursing article written more than three decades ago uses the phrase *professional intimacy* to indicate the resolved stage of role confusion for nurses who are transitioning from the bedside to nurse practitioner (post-undergraduate work).[18] Although it suggests that nurses and doctors mutually depend on each other in a professionally intimate manner, this article does not specifically define professional intimacy; nor does it address the work bedside nurses do with patients.

In this book, I use the phrase *professional intimacy* to name the theoretical model I designed after conducting research with bedside nurses at associate and bachelor levels of nursing education. I define professional intimacy as the set of intimate exchanges among nurses, patients, and family members through which the nurse must balance the patient's emotional and physical needs in a turbulent work environment. I explicitly choose the word *intimacy* rather than the word *care* to mark this labor because doing so makes clear that we are talking about work conditions as exchanges that are socially defined as private.[19] Moreover, I distinguish intimacy from other parts of care and explain that professional intimacy is one part of the science of nursing care. Using the word *professional* along with *intimacy* unabashedly claims that intimacy in the context of hospital nursing is professional labor.

I analyze intimate care in the context of hospital nursing not as a natural attribute but as a routine pattern. When nurses and other people define care as a natural ability, they mask the skill and knowledge needed to make intimate labor *seem* natural. I highlight intimate trust strategies in part to demonstrate *how* some nurses can make care seem natural through the provision of care that is simultaneously professional and intimate.[20] Professional intimacy encompasses more than physical, emotional, and intimate connections. Professional intimacy is work that requires skill, experience, and strategy. Professional intimacy articulates the complex set of interactions nurses perform to build and maintain trust with their patients so patients can receive optimal health care. Throughout this research, I found that nurses professionally and intimately negotiated a cycle of trust, conflict, and renewed trust with their patients to ensure quality care (see Appendix C for a diagram of professional intimacy). When patients entered the hospital, they experienced a range of feelings. Some patients felt hope and trusted their nurses immediately. With these patients, I watched nurses make the most of this trust through a series of strategic interactions that helped to further facilitate a sense of intimacy that developed this trust. Other patients felt fear and other negative feelings upon entering the hospital. I watched nurses work through conflicts and establish trust with these patients.

I center my discussion on intimate conditions in health care in part to show how the process of giving and receiving quality health care can *begin* in conflict because many patients enter the hospital already feeling fear and a lack of trust of the medical and health-care industries. Patients' mistrust of doctors and nurses is underemphasized in general discussions about nursing and, if discussed at all, is not posited as a condition of receiving health care but, rather, as a special circumstance of some patients. As soon as nurses encountered their patients, I watched them provide intimate labor to create trust, negotiate conflict, and renew trust to ensure quality health care.

I found that how nurses established trust sometimes caused conflict because patients felt overentitled to intimacy and acted out in verbally, physically, and emotionally abusive ways. Unlike workers in many other jobs, who can readily report such behaviors to management, nurses alleviated these conflicts so patients could again feel trust and regain comfort and confidence. Nurses turned to their strategies of professional intimacy to alleviate conflict and reestablish trust, and these strategies changed according to intersections of race, gender, and nationality. It is this trust work that fostered the accomplishment of quality health care. Without it, patients and/or their families were less likely to cooperate in their health care. Because nurses must be sure patients trust them to provide quality care, they need education, training, and a specific knowledge set regarding how to negotiate intimacy in a professional setting.

My aim in discussing professional intimacy is to offer a framework that combines the intimate with professional life, which changes according to perceptions and constructions of social identities. As a model, professional intimacy provides a language for patients, nurses, and administrators to explain, teach, conduct, and advocate for knowledgeable and skilled intimate care in a hospital setting. My goal is the inclusion of best-practices training as a result of this analysis in nursing school and places of employment. This would better nurses' labor conditions and increase public understandings of care. My study has significant implications for the health-care crisis because it examines the relationships among commercialized intimacy; the work conditions of nurses; and the effects of gender, race, and nationality. Moreover, it implies that care—as a social and economic act—changes meaning according to social context. In this book, I argue that if care occurs in context, then we must let go of ideas that some nurses are naturally better at caring than others; that some nurses are "born to care"; or that nursing is a gift, a sacrifice, or a calling.

Intersectionality Theory

Anna was one of several Latina nurses in my study. She was born in the United States after her parents had emigrated from Mexico. She spoke both Spanish and English fluently with a slight Spanish accent. She was also brown-skinned. These factors in combination contributed to how Anna experienced her work conditions. They shaped how and when patients trusted her in the health-care process. Alan and Maura disbelieved Anna's role as Alan's nurse, despite her introduction of herself to them as his nurse and her efforts as a professional caregiver. Many researchers have documented historical and contemporary workplace discrimination against immigrant and nonimmigrant women of color in care and service work.[21] Some of these researchers have specifically documented discrimination within nursing and detailed how women of color are viewed as unprofessional and white women are viewed as professional.[22]

Just as falsely relating care and naturalness hides the skill of intimate trust strategies, it also minimizes how social categories such as race, gender, and nationality contribute to ideas that make intimate labor seem, on the one hand, either unnatural or natural and, on the other hand, either professional or unprofessional. Hospital administrators told me they expected nurses to care equally for each patient, but nurses said, and my observations verified, that patients reacted differently depending on how they perceived their nurse's race, gender, and nationality. Patients treated white women and white men as professionals and treated women of color[23] as ultracaring but also unskilled.[24] Patients and administrators tended not to expect white men to be nurturing, and administrators encouraged them to advance away from the bedside and into supervisory positions because they thought men would be better leaders than women.[25] It is important to note that this "glass escalator"[26] excluded men of color.[27]

Intersectionality is a conceptual and methodological framework that explains how discrete social categories—for example, race, gender, sexuality, class, and nationality—work together to create unique experiences of privilege and subordination in everyday life. In 1989, renowned legal theorist Kimberlé Crenshaw coined the term *intersectionality* to explain the unique sexual harassments experienced by women of color, which often include simultaneous racist and sexist interactions:

> I wish that everyone could have heard the story of an Asian construction worker whose co-workers shoved a hammer between her legs, who was taunted with racial slurs, who was repeatedly grabbed on her breasts while installing overhead fixtures, and who was asked whether it was true that Asian women's vaginas were sideways. She testified that when she was told, "you don't belong here," she couldn't figure out whether it was because she was Asian, Female or both.[28]

Crenshaw argues that legal and everyday definitions of sexual harassment as gender discrimination do not discuss how the experience of, and consequences for, sexual harassment are constructed by both racism and sexism.[29] If law-yers (and by extension scholars, activists, and employers) prioritize gender when defining what is and what is not sexual harassment, many experiences of women of color get lost. In her analysis of court cases, legal theorist The-resa Beiner makes this very point.[30] Beiner demonstrates that judges, when presented in court with harassment cases that contain both sexual and racial elements, toss these cases because they do not fit within existing legal frames.

In this study, I use the intersectional approach to analyze intimate care work from the perspective of nurses who are diverse by race, gender, and nationality and who care for patients who are also diverse by these identities. As a result, this book shows how intersectionality better articulates the expe-riences and perceptions of the nurses in my study, because nurses perceive that the intimate care they provide to patients changes at the intersections of race, gender, and nationality. My analysis responds to Patricia Hill Collins's call to use intersectionality to study social life and Kimberlé Crenshaw and Bonnie Thorton Dill's mandate to include race and ethnicity in applications of intersectionality.[31]

Throughout the book, I demonstrate how intersectionality is essential to the conceptualization of professional intimacy. Intersectionality informs the process of professional intimacy, and professional intimacy demonstrates how to use the intersectional approach.[32] In fact, without intersectionality, I could not have conceptualized professional intimacy as it is explained in this book. Intersectionality theory is integral to the concept of professional intimacy because it helps speak on behalf of all nurses and patients who live at intersections of racial, gendered, and national identities. This analysis also demonstrates how to use intersectionality as an analytic to assess, measure, and articulate professionally intimate care work.

The intersectional approach offers an epistemological change in care by explaining both exploitative and potentially emancipatory caring arrange-ments at the social and economic site of intimate care in nursing. Rather than define care as a personality trait that some individuals possess, this analysis reveals that "to be caring" is a social act that changes at the structural and ideological intersections of race, gender, and nationality. Because it focuses on structural conditions of life and not on individual personality attributes, the intersectional approach helps take the responsibility from the natural abilities of individuals and places it on the ways that social patterns influence indi-viduals' behaviors and interactions with each other. This method also helps clearly acknowledge the increasing diversity in nursing and shows how the labor of nurses is constructed by these and other intersections. The intersec-tional approach helps define professional intimacy in terms that incorporate the intersections of gender, race, and nationality to recognize the diverse work experiences of nurses and the diverse meanings of quality health care.

Commercialized and Commodified Intimacies

When Anna asserted a professional boundary with Alan, he responded with a sexual innuendo. Alan's remark that Anna "could make it up to him" when she said he could not talk to her in a racist-sexist manner could be read as innocent, even playful. Yet, as explained throughout this book, his words represent a consistent pattern in sexualized interactions, which nurses had to negotiate in order to give their patients care. I observed nurses negotiate sexualized intimacy in many forms: as patients' physical and verbal advances and as patients' sexual intimacy with a visitor.

Anna and many others, especially new nurses, told me they sometimes could not respond to sexualized advances and insults from patients, for several reasons. First, they did not feel prepared to handle such interactions from someone they felt was dependent on them for care. They were trained as professionals, and it did not occur to them that patients would ever behave in a sexual manner while in the hospital. Second, some nurses felt there was no institutional recourse or support for their experiences because they did not feel that these behaviors coming from patients counted as sexual harassment. Finally, many nurses shouldered the burden of their experiences alone because they thought that they should be able to handle all patient interactions as part of their individual practice. They feared that if they sought help for these situations, they would appear incompetent.

I analyze these sexualized interactions from patients in the context of literature on commercialized and commodified intimacies as part of the labor process.[33] Although the two are often conflated, *commercialized intimacy* involves the process (i.e., business methods and strategies) of gaining profit from intimacy, and *commodified intimacy* refers to intimacy that is for sale when it was not once before. Intimacy alone is a feeling or an experience. Commodified intimacy is a product that can be bought and sold. Commercialized intimacies describe this market exchange: the marketing, the selling, the buying, and the investing of intimacy as part of labor or as part of industry.

In a recent collection devoted to various types of commercialized intimate labors, Viviana Zelizer, a renowned scholar of the relationship between the economic and the intimate, frames the occurrence of intimacy in labor three ways: as unpaid care in intimate settings, as unpaid care in economic organizations, and as paid care in intimate settings.[34] Zelizer focuses on the economic value of unpaid care in homes and other private spaces, the threat and potential of intimacy in corporations and other economic organizations, and the governmental compensation to individuals who provide care for people in household-based care.[35] By her own admission, Zelizer avoids discussion "of paid care in economic organizations on the ground that we already know more about the varieties of care provided by medical professionals and other licensed caregivers than we do about caring elsewhere."[36] She is quick to add, however, "Even there we can gain a clearer understanding through recognition that, in the delivery of care, professionals and their clients are likewise negotiating definitions of their social relations and forms of compensation to represent those definitions."[37] I also assert that the work of hospital nurses in particular is important to the examination of social and economic relations of intimacy, because nurses provide paid care in an economic organization (hospital) and also in a household-like arrangement (the patient's room).

The study of commercialized intimacy reveals how sex, care, and emotions including love are bought and sold in the market as products. These exchanges include how intimacy is the product, as in the case of sex work, care work, and other jobs that require workers to produce intimacy in direct exchange for compensation.[38] These exchanges also include those in a work environment that is sexualized to increase profit or how formerly nonsexual work environments become sexualized as part of employee interactions, as in the cases of feminist magazine production, taxicab drivers, and restaurant work.[39] These exchanges can also include sexual harassment from customers that is common, part of the job, and sometimes institutionalized as in the case of waitress work.[40]

Although Anna did not receive direct compensation for providing intimate care to Alan, I observed a pattern over time in which patients and family members gave "tips" to nurses in appreciation for their care. Patients and family members expressed their gratitude to nurses by giving stuffed animals, flowers, and candy. Some nurses told me that patients also offered money to thank them for their service. In addition, although actual hospitals are quite opposite from a sexualized workplace, hospitals and nurses are represented as "sexy" on television and in film. Nursing scholars argue that these representations could affect the work conditions of actual nurses.[41] Finally, most of the nurses did not speak about sexualized interactions as sexual harassment, and senior nurses acknowledged that these interactions felt like "part of the job."[42]

None of my observations about commercialized intimate labors throughout my study quite explain the interaction between Anna and Alan, as Anna described it to me. She did not receive a tip from Alan; nor did she feel that her workplace was sexualized or that comments like Alan's could be a regular part of her job. Nevertheless, this interaction contained commercialized intimate labor because Anna had performed emotional and body labor as part of her nursing care for Alan. The study of commercialized intimate labor includes emotional and body labor as defined by how corporations make demands on, and profit off of, the emotions and bodies of workers.[43] In her landmark study of flight attendants in the United States, Arlie Russell Hochschild coined the phrase *emotional labor* to explain how employers appropriate the emotions of workers and make this a condition of their employees' labor to ensure customer satisfaction and accumulate profit.[44] Hochschild states that not all jobs that involve care include emotional labor. She explains that the jobs that do include emotional labor have three common characteristics: "First, they require face-to-face or voice-to-voice contact with the public. Second, they require the worker to produce an emotional state in another person—gratitude or fear, for example. Third, they allow the employer, through training and supervision, to exercise a degree of control over the emotional activities of employees."[45] This last feature could exclude nurses from Hochschild's conception of emotional workers. As professional care workers, nurses have significant autonomy over their work with patients and do not experience the same degree of control by administrators as other workers described by Hochschild. Nurses manage their own interactions with individual patients, and supervisors do not insist on controlling these individualized interactions.[46] Nurses are, however, managed by an industry that in large part defines care through the feelings it produces in patients. At the same time, nurses strategically negotiate emotions, bodies, and intimate behaviors as part of their labor. I observed, however, that experienced nurses knew that establishing intimacy, negotiating the conflict that sometimes results from that intimacy, and reestablishing intimacy results in quality health care and patient satisfaction.

Hochschild distinguished emotional labor from individual uses of emotion in social interaction by drawing on the work of sociologists Emile Durkheim and Erving Goffman. She explains that the use of emotion in social interaction includes how individuals manage their own emotions to avoid interpersonal conflict. Emotions affect customs, too; they help encourage proper behavior and maintain social order. Emotional labor is different from these uses of feelings because corporations purposefully manipulate and exploit the feelings of workers to make money. Emotional labor alienates workers from their "true selves," which prohibits possibilities for worker resistance to unfair work conditions.

For more than two decades, scholars have confirmed Hochschild's theory of emotional labor and expanded it to include employee negotiation of emotions and resistance to employer dominance.[47] Institutions obligate individual nurses to provide "quality" care under any and all circumstances. Patients feel entitled to "quality" care in part because they need it but also because they *pay* for it. In both situations, what quality care means is unclear. British nursing scholar Nicky James uses emotional labor to discuss the "ambivalent status" and exploitative features of care in nursing.[48] Since James, other scholars have identified how nurses negotiate boundaries with their patients[49] and increase patient comfort[50] by actively adjusting their presentations of self through their demeanors and facial expressions.

Professional intimacy differs from emotional and body labor in part because nurses chose to do this work knowing it would lead to better care—not because they or their company would make more money. Hochschild conceptualized emotional labor to articulate how employers require workers to use their own emotions to increase corporate profit. Unlike emotional labor as Hochschild conceptualized it, professional intimacy is not a strategy of the employer to increase hospital profit; rather, it is a strategy nurses employ to perform their jobs effectively. Emotional labor is one aspect of professional intimacy because it explains how nurses' emotional labor is exploited if left unnoticed by the health-care industry, but it does not fully explain intimate care in nursing because it is not a mandate by the hospital administration.

Commercialized intimacy in labor is part of the increasing commodification of intimacy that permeates and sustains global capitalism.[51] This is to say that as our society advances economically, culturally, and technologically, intimacy and capital become more tightly linked.[52] The commodification of intimacy reveals the connections between micro-level interactions such as those between nurses and patients and macro-level processes such as the relationship between the nursing shortage and the global economy.[53] It shows how experiences of the intimate construct social relations and how social relations such as those that are race-based or gender-oriented construct intimate experiences. To make these connections between micro and macro analyses of intimacy, I again draw on the work of sociologist Viviana Zelizer. Zelizer shows how intimacy is bought and sold not just as products or labor but as part of everyday interactions.

In *The Purchase of Intimacy*, Zelizer challenges readers to avoid separating economic life from the intimate, since intimacy is often framed as too soft, too feminine, or too sexual to be taken seriously by economists and other storytellers of public life.[54] Instead, Zelizer emphasizes the combination of intimacy and economics that are seen in divorce obligations, struggles for the rights of same-sex couples, and professional and unpaid care work. Zelizer argues that money does not necessarily degrade intimate activity and, more relevant to nursing, that the work of intimate care does not make economic activity inefficient. She suggests it is the "grip"—the resilience—of intimacy that makes it a necessary part of economic exchange. Even though the nurses I studied were overrun balancing multiple technical, administrative, and medical tasks, they displayed significant compassion when caring for patients and families. In Zelizer's words, they "employ the skilled practices of personal intimacy—joking, cajoling, consoling, and sympathetic listening."[55] This "resilience of intimacy" in nursing helps patients and family members receive quality health care.

Nurses have fought a long battle to be taken seriously in the medical industry. Framing nursing as professional labor has been an important part of this effort. However, it is this same professionalization that reduces the value of intimate care work. Zelizer demonstrates how "professional organizations, courts, and legislatures collaborate in protecting the boundary of professional practice."[56] First, professional organizations worry about the corruption of professional practice, and second, they fear that a focus on intimacy will promote unwanted intimacies. For example, lap dancing laws distinguish prostitution from exotic dancing by setting rules about access between dancers and customers. I found this sort of concern in my research as well. Nurses feared that any discussion of intimacy would take away from the professionalism in nursing work and would also promote an inappropriate sexualization of relationships in professional care.

In this book, I show how professionally intimate care work fits into the larger system of commercialized and commodified intimacies because it seems especially pertinent to several questions about the contemporary state of nursing in the United States and, more generally, about meanings of commercialized and commodified intimacy in professional work. The book addresses how and why new nurses seem unprepared to handle intimacy, in spite of their training, when compared to experienced nurses. Further, it provides one reason why large numbers of experienced nurses leave the bedside and take administrative roles or leave the profession altogether. The book demonstrates how nurses, administrators, and patients idealize care, which only serves to reinforce the misunderstanding of this labor. It reveals the triple bind of professionalism, technical skill, and care expectations that reduces the job of nursing to categories that cannot reflect the complex and intimate strategies nurses use every day to care for their patients. It challenges the idea that there is one standard way to care and that one either does or does not have this "gift." Most importantly, it reveals that although compassion as a personality trait can seem natural to individual people, care as professional knowledge can be, should be, and *is* consistently taught to nurses. Administrative recognition of professionally intimate labor as something to be articulated, taught, and formally counted as nurses' work would improve the work conditions of nurses because it would help make space and time for this labor, which is an element critical to patients' health and satisfaction.

Outline of the Book

The rest of this book is organized into Chapters 1 to 5 and the Conclusion. In Chapter 1, I discuss the fact that nurse directors and hospital administrators greatly valued care but could not articulate how care occurred and did not believe it could be taught. I also explore their avoidance of the word *intimacy* when describing nursing. I suggest that the failure to recognize intimacy is at the core of misunderstanding the process of care. Many nurses, patients, and administrators see acts of care through what might best be described as a Florence Nightingale lens: natural to women and indicative of pure and altruistic motives.[57] Contemporary "Florence Nightingales" glorify care in nursing from what used to be considered a religious calling and is now described as a moral imperative.[58] This rhetoric could increase the social value of caregiving, but it actually reinforces gender stereotypes of women as natural and preferred caregivers and care as a personal attribute rather than as professional knowledge.[59] I bring in my data and other studies on male nurses to challenge the natural relationship between femininity and care. I show how administrators seem to contradict themselves when they want a naturally caring nurse for a job that is professional.

In Chapter 2, I draw on sociology of gender and intimacy theories to help conceptualize how being a caring nurse is not a natural personality characteristic but is in fact work that includes managing conflict, is inextricably linked to money, and changes depending on the specific social interaction and according to social and economic forces. I distinguish between personal identity and identities as social constructs to introduce how I use the intersectional approach. I then explain the intersectional approach in more detail and connect it to the salient intersections in my study: those of gender, race, and nationality. In the second part of the chapter, I connect my study to the global enterprise of care by introducing the relationship between professional intimacy and the nursing shortage. I draw on theories of emotional labor, body labor, and intimacy as purchase to show how administrators misunderstand the intentions of nurses and how everyone in the hospital contributes to a consumer culture of patient satisfaction. These explanations serve as an important backdrop to my findings on how nurses develop and sustain intimate trust with patients.

Chapter 3 describes the first stage of professional intimacy: how nurses build, negotiate, and sustain what I call *intimate trust* with their patients. I discuss how bedside nurses described the value of intimacy in nursing care. Nurses did not feel their labor was intimate, but knew that intimacy was important to the patient. This finding helps answer the question about how nurses can both value and reject intimacy in their work. I explain what I call *intimate conflict* in Chapter 4. I found, through my observations and nurses' interpretations of these observations, that relaxed boundaries and a sense of entitlement sometimes encouraged patients to express anger and sexual desire toward nurses. As a result, nurses felt and negotiated discomfort, tension, and threat. Chapter 5 explains how nurses created boundaries that addressed intimate conflict while maintaining intimate trust with patients and family members. I also explain why and how nurses were pressured to handle intimate conflict on their own. As a corrective to this approach, I emphasize the benefits of what I call *collective intimacy* as a strategy for dealing with these conflicts.

In the Conclusion, I turn my attention to theoretical and practical uses of this book. Theoretically speaking, I hope that this model of professional intimacy contributes to understanding of the relationship between commercialized intimacies and the global economy. I also hope that it serves to model how the intersectional approach can be used to study everyday meanings of care. In addition, this model could be tested and developed to help explain intimate labor in other professions. Practically speaking, hospital nursing care and nursing education might be restructured to better accommodate professional intimacy. Hospitals that institutionally and collectively recognize professional intimacy would help nurses better understand the shared conditions of their labor. Attention to issues of professional intimacy in nurse training and in hospitals would also increase nurse retention and patient satisfaction, which could help alleviate the nursing shortage. Professional intimacy demonstrates the significance of both professionalism and intimate labor in nursing practices. As a model and labor practice, it rejects dichotomous framings of care as either altruism or professional skill and demonstrates how hospital nurses use both to provide quality care to patients and families. This book reframes the discussion of what it means to be a good nurse by rejecting traditional definitions of care, femininity, and whiteness. Rather than focus on whether nurses are motivated to care for either altruistic or economic reasons, this book shows that nurses and patients construct what it means to provide care along intersections of race, gender, and nationality.

1

Invisible Intimacy in Nursing

No administrator at the hospital could articulate the process of care—for example, how nurses specifically made patients feel safe or responded to their needs across many different contexts. This did not mean that hospital leaders did not value care. The hospital demonstrated the priority it placed on care through its mission, its value statements, and its Magnet status. While all three of these acknowledged care in various ways, none of them included topics related to professional intimacy. For example, my interview with the hospital president revealed that, although he valued nurses, he could not say how care happened and could not acknowledge the expertise needed to negotiate intimacy. He said, "I don't know how they do it. I am just grateful they do!" On the surface, the president's sentiments seem to express his appreciation for nurses and even, perhaps, his support of their work. On a deeper level, these sentiments mask the actual work he appreciates. The hospital president expressed gratitude for the nurses' ability to handle intimate care but for what exact skills, he did not know. He values care but does so in a way that mythologizes it and hides intimate labor practices.

These findings from my interview with the hospital president mirror what I observed at the hospital, where staff and administration alike effused about the importance of care but no one identified its meaning or acknowledged the practice of intimate labor. Consider this statement that describes the hospital's work culture: "Mutual respect and care are the underpinnings of our culture. They create a work environment where everyone feels valued and appreciated, where employees look forward to going to work every day."[1] What does it mean for "mutual respect and care" to facilitate "a work environment where everyone feels valued and appreciated"? Mutual respect and care are the subjects of this sentence, but respect and care do not just happen. Framing care this way makes the intimate aspects of nurses' care work invisible. The statement expresses what I witnessed as genuinely held values at the hospital, but it fails to recognize how this environment is achieved on any practical level.

The hospital also demonstrated its commitment to care by including in its nursing literature statements such as "_____ Hospital always cares for you" and "The staff are true professionals who sincerely care about the patients and each other." Here nurses are identified as professional, but care is broadly described as a value or a feeling one may experience upon entering the hospital doors. Instead of marking intimate labor as distinct from other forms of care, these statements conflate various types of care: medical care, technical care, care coordination (care plans), personal care, and of course, care as a way of being—a way of being "nice."

To be taken seriously by the medical profession, nurses emphasized measurable outcomes of their labor, such as technical and medical care. They partitioned care as a value separate from professional labor. They found care difficult to describe and also used it as a lump-sum term to refer to various aspects of nursing. Consider the following quotation from a nurse administrator when I asked her to define different aspects of care:

> I think it would be very difficult, and the reason I say that is, oh, the technical would outweigh the professional. But not really, because really, what's happening at the same time is that the nurse is thinking, and that's the distinction of a professional—is thinking while performing the technical. So, I might be giving a patient a medication, and there's the technical part, the robot part when I go over and get the medication and I look at the record of how much I should give, and I walk it to the patient's room. But the professional side, of evaluating the patient's allergies, what are the other medications that the patient's on, what has the response to the medication been, and then if I think they're going to go home on it, teaching them about this at the same time that I'm administering it. It's difficult to separate it out.

It is important to note that this administrator began her response by saying it would be difficult to define different aspects of care. She was not alone.

Although I observed nurses distinguish different aspects of their care labor through their actions with patients and sometimes in their communications with each other, they did not formally discern these aspects on reports or in case notes. Instead, nurses and administrators either used the word *care* to talk about all aspects—intimate, professional, or technical—or they did as this administrator did: they emphasized technical and professional work and ignored care as a labor process.

Many administrators and some nurses could not partition different types of nursing care outside of the technical and medical and instead used one word, *care*, to mean it all. In contrast, I read documentation that distinguished some care tasks from others. Consider how care responsibilities are articulated as "coordinating care, monitoring care, educating patients about care, and providing excellent care" in a job advertisement for a nurse: "Coordinates patient care . . . evaluates effectiveness of care provided by comparing patient response with observable outcomes . . . [i]dentifies and delivers initial and ongoing patient/family's education needs as an integral part of care delivery . . . provides excellent patient care." Unlike the language that conflates meanings of care, this advertisement distinguished between care as something nurses measured and care as something nurses provided. The beginning of this advertisement identified various care tasks: coordinate care, monitor patient response, and educate families and patients. Here the focus of care was on activities that are observable and measurable. The last requirement was to "provide excellent care," but I was unsure what that could mean. What did nurses do to make sure care was "excellent"? Were they just naturally nice? Were they serene? What if the patient refused care? How did they know they had done this part of their job? Was there a "provides excellent care" checklist? For the first care responsibilities, there were checklists and charts to be sure this work was accomplished. There were no such types of accountability for the last care responsibility. How to "provide excellent care" seemed to depend on a nurse's individual discretion.

To practice something, one needs to know it exists. While experienced bedside nurses discussed the importance of intimacy in their work, hospital administrators (who were also trained nurses) denied its existence. No one spoke of intimacy and none of the recognition programs, incentive programs, work policies, or work procedures mentioned intimacy in any way. The word *intimacy* was essentially absent from hospital institutional culture. There was no mention of intimacy in any conversation I observed at staff meetings or other workplace meetings. I did not see any reference to intimacy in documented care policy or procedure. In hospital nursing care, intimacy was invisible. Consider the following exchange with Anita, a unit director. I tried to understand if and how she noticed how her staff negotiated intimacy with patients:

> LISA: How do you determine productive intimacy? When is it success-ful? How do you distinguish it from uncomfortable interactions?
>
> ANITA: Now, are you asking me personally, or how do I judge my staff?
>
> LISA: Both from you. Break it up. Personally first or however you want to answer.
>
> ANITA: Okay, so how—what's the question again?
>
> LISA: How do you determine that intimate touching is promoting healing?
>
> ANITA: Okay, I remember going to—every so often I'd do patient in-terviews and, ah, I mean, and I'm in there talking to a little man or a little lady. It's so easy to just take their hand. I mean, you can see them just either relaxed by how their face—and, you know, it's the right thing that you're doing. Um, so I—I think that that's acceptable.

Rather than talk about her staff, Anita responded with a story about when, as a young nurse, she discovered she felt a nonsexual, intimate con-nection to a young male patient. I remember vividly how Anita struggled with the question about intimacy as I imagined her sorting through different meanings of intimacies in her mind. "Was it personal intimacy?" she may have wondered. "No, it's about my staff. She wants to know how we assess intimacy," she may have thought. Instead of talking about how she assesses nurses, I watched her search through her mind to find the words to explain how she is professionally intimate with her patients. I remember the look on her face when she did not have the words to describe what she later told me was paramount to quality health care.

At the end of the interview, Anita said that nurses should talk more about intimacy but that they never will:

> I think some discussions like this should happen, like in nursing schools. I mean, they never will—they never do. I mean, on a normal case, you—I'm going to guess that they don't happen over—there's so much [to learn], I guess. And of course, there's so much technical knowledge to learn that—and I don't think that even though nurses are in an intimate, uh, spot with their . . . patients, that's something that we always are comfortable confronting. Like, we don't usually talk to each other about this kind of stuff at all. Yeah, we don't. [*Laughs.*]

In my conversation with Anita, I first asked her questions that might help her locate the professionalism of intimate care that I observed her nurses engage in every day. Instead, Anita struggled to find language to explain how she professionally handled intimacy as a bedside nurse. Anita remarked how intimacy should be discussed in nursing school, but she seemed skeptical. She suggested that perhaps intimacy would not be discussed in nursing school because of the amount of knowledge nurses need to learn now. She quickly admitted, however, that it was likely that intimacy would not be talked about because nurses were uncomfortable with the idea of intimacy. Perhaps this discussion would be easier if nurses shared that intimacy could be private and public; personal and professional. Intimacy contributes to quality health care even if it is something that is difficult to measure and articulate.

I think this failure to recognize intimacy as valid labor is at the core of misunderstandings of the various aspects of care and their roles in nursing work.[2] Intimate care is invisible in nursing practice and nursing education because providing this kind of care is a process, not an outcome, and as a process care is defined as something that is natural, not something that is measurable. If asked, nurses can show patients, families, and their supervisors how much medicine they have administered to a patient. They can document the number and type of referrals they give. They can quantify bodily fluids. They cannot, however, explain how they *provide intimate care* and perhaps more importantly how this aspect of caring is critical to a patient's well-being and to quality health care in general. Instead, they discuss bedside care as a natural personality characteristic or as a moral calling.

There are several costs to glorifying care as a universal attribute or ethic. First, when we glorify care as natural we exclude "regular" people, those people who do not identify as natural caregivers but could potentially become successful nurses. Regular people include all those people who were not "born" to care, such as individuals who enter nursing after changing careers. Excluding regular people from nursing negatively affects nurse recruitment. Second, when we glorify care as a universal attribute, we more easily blame individual nurses when care goes wrong. If a patient is unhappy or if caring for patients is not easy for a new nurse, it must be the fault of the new nurse, not her work conditions. Internalizing an apparent inability to care while simultaneously not knowing how to cope with the stress of providing professionally intimate care will contribute to new nurse burnout, which negatively affects nurse retention. Third, when we falsely naturalize intimate care, we eliminate the "professional" in professional care work because it erases the need for education, training, skill, knowledge, and practice. Naturalizing intimate care as a gift, sacrifice, or ethical imperative exacerbates the invisibility of care work because it removes the focus from the labor of caring by emphasizing the belief that all individuals should care because it is the right thing to do. It defines intimate care as ethical outcomes rather than as professional and laborious practices. Naturalizing and glorifying care contributes to the invisibility of the skill and knowledge required for intimacy in care and the professional labor that makes providing this care *look* natural.

Care as a Natural Personality Trait

In our interview, Anita could not recall nurses taking classes on intimacy. She said: "We didn't have classes on or even asked us if we were uncomfortable touching patients or anything like that. I think that was like a given. I mean, I don't even remember anyone asking me how I even felt about it, or anything. I didn't feel uncomfortable but I don't think that it ever came up."

When intimacy did come up in my study, nurses talked about it as important care work that stems from their natural emotions. As one administrator put it when I asked her about how nurses manage emotions in care, "It affects it a great deal, actually. First, as a nurse for many years myself, I'm aware of the emotional aspect of giving care. [It is] both the part of joy and happiness as well as some of the most difficult times that people face." What this administrator did not say is that nurses and administrators rarely talked about intimacy as a pattern of care and instead drew on how good nurses were naturally adept at managing emotions, using phrases like "personal energy" and "intrinsic desire."[3] Consider the following quotation from Dawn, a nursing educator, as she explains how care is something nurses naturally bring to the workplace:

> I don't think people who enter the profession [would] if they didn't have that intrinsic desire, I guess to care, or understand a little bit about it, and then they probably wouldn't choose it [nursing]. But then it goes back to how you would define that. We all learn caring from, you know, the knowledge that we pick up as a child or the actions or behaviors that we see, so I guess the action of caring is different than the actual definition of what that is, you know, and how you operationalize it, I guess. It's something that you pick up on the job.

It is noteworthy that Dawn initially said nurses bring care to the job and then said that care is "something that is picked up" there. This, and other contradictions like it, suggested to me that perhaps "how to do care" can be taught—if we can articulate how and when it is labor. For those who feel caring comes naturally to them, this would make them better able to explain and develop their caring skills. Further, given the nursing shortage and the overall need for jobs in a struggling national economy, it seems likely that individuals would choose nursing whether or not they have had a "calling." This means that individuals who do not necessarily identify as naturally caring could choose to be a nurse and execute the mandate to care effectively.

Of course, this education is not currently taking place. Dawn's statement supports my concern that *how* nurses intimately care is confusing and invisible in nursing education. That intimacy is invisible in descriptions of care keeps the focus on how being caring is a natural personality trait. These ideas sustain the belief that intimate care cannot be taught in nursing school. Consider the following passage from a university nursing professor I interviewed:

> Well, my own feeling is we don't teach caring. I think that we couldn't. We could probably break it down into a scale, but at the end of the program, they [undergraduate students] take a test and the test is not based on caring. The test is based on skills. It's based on assessment skill, diagnosing skills, planning skills. Now, a piece of that in there is probably caring, but we don't test that. What kind of a nursing diagnosis would you give to them [students] rather than the physical assessment skills? How do you assess that emotional interaction between the people?

This nursing professor was stumped by how she would assess a student's ability to care. As she said, nursing students are tested on their skills, not on their care. She implied that care is not a skill because it is not testable and that care is not testable because it is not a skill. This tautological thinking keeps intimacy in care invisible and makes care seem natural because care that is natural to a person cannot be assessed.

Care, in this sense, is purely subjective. Can you explain why one individual seems more caring than another? How do you define care? We cannot explain how one person is nicer than the first. The person just *is* nice. It is part of her. It is a part of her being. It is natural to her makeup. This person does not have to work to be nice; she simply is so. Most of us tend to define care as synonymous with niceness. Renowned nursing advocate and writer Suzanne Gordon found that patients assess good nurses as natural caregivers, those who are gentle, kind, and attentive. When patients write memoirs about their illnesses, most focus on the role of nurses with a gift for being nice, rather than as knowledgeable medical providers.[4] This separation of skill and care reinforces the idea that caring well can be attributed to one's natural personality, not work that is taught and learned over time.

Conventional definitions of femininity influence the relationship between care and niceness by obscuring how care is work. In her book *Nursing against the Odds*, Gordon describes how nurses and the general public view Florence Nightingale as the ideal nurse, an angel of mercy who is naturally compassionate and kind to her patients. When news journalists fail to describe nursing as a thriving profession filled with images of skilled and compassionate nurses, they revert to the image of Florence Nightingale carrying a lamp or create cartoon characters of women nurses with angel wings. Interestingly, the angel of mercy image is in stark contrast to the actual Florence Nightingale, who actually crusaded for better work conditions for nurses, rather than for nurses to be inherently good individuals or, the reverse, for inherently good individuals to become nurses.

There is a relationship between the idea of a good nurse and ideas of traditional femininity. Traditional femininity, and, by extension, nursing, are defined as pleasing others. Care—whether an act or idea—is about pleasing others. Florence Nightingale—an advocate for safe patient care and improved working conditions for nurses—became the icon of the naturally caring nurse, the lady with the lamp, and the angel of mercy because nursing is a job that is linked specifically with natural traits conventionally associated with femininity. Gordon explains, "Perhaps because contemporary nursing has been so closely associated with traditional femininity, no feminist biographer has taken on the historical challenge of examining how patriarchal iconography tamed Nightingale, transforming a tough, acerbic, and complicated woman into a Victorian angel of mercy."[5] Ideas of what it means to be truly feminine helped to "tame" Florence Nightingale as an ideal woman. Before 1870 nurses did not receive formal training for their work. Instead, women who nursed their own families to health or were former patients themselves became nurses.[6] Becoming a nurse seemed like a natural move for women, especially in a time that idealized women as naturally (i.e., biologically) more domestic, submissive, pious, and pure than men. Historian Barbara Welter first conceptualized these social ideals as the cult of true womanhood.[7]

The cult of true womanhood explains how regardless of the actual racial, sexual, and classed conditions of women's lives, a social ideology persisted that helped define normal femininity. This meant that women were pressured to look a certain way, act a certain way, and believe in certain values to be considered "real" women in society. If a woman did not meet these expectations, she suffered social stigma, rejection, and violence. Women were publicly accepted as women if they possessed what were defined as natural virtues: domesticity, purity, piety, and submissiveness to men. This meant that women possessed the natural ability to clean and care, and these abilities are what brought them closest to God. As Welter argues, there was a clear relationship between women's subordination and women's natural ability to care. Welter also explained that the cult of true womanhood was constructed by race and class. That is, women of color and working and poor women were automatically exempted from this ideology because it was imagined through the lens of white and middle-class society. As a social ideology, the cult of true womanhood shaped middle-class white women's experiences and also helped to justify racism, heterosexism, and an economic system that idealized white men as paid workers and located white women in the home.

The cult of true womanhood helps us consider the intersecting roles of gender and race in dominant conceptions of care as natural. As a social ideology, whiteness traditionally acquires meanings of purity, goodness, and innocence, becoming a category against which other racial experiences are judged deficient.[8] Whiteness as a social construct contributes to the Florence Nightingale image of nurse because it helps to formulate the expectation that true nurses, the kind that are angels of mercy, are white. Most media and other controlling images depict nurses as white women who graciously, easily, and professionally provide care to patients.[9] This image of the dominant nurse is at the intersection of race (whiteness), nationality (English-speaking) and gender (femininity). This intersection defines "true" nursing care as pure, selfless, and professionally effortless.

Although white women constitute the majority of degreed and licensed nurses in the United States, Australia, Great Britain, and other Western nations, the numbers of men and women of color working in the U.S. nursing industry have increased in recent years.[10] Their work, however, is not positioned in the same way as the work of white women nurses. Typically, when women of color provide paid care work, it is either invisible or superficially glorified as extra-natural and unprofessional when compared to care work provided by white women.[11] Sociologist Pierrette Hondagneu-Sotelo is one of several scholars who have examined how U.S. employers of immigrant Latina domestic workers view domestic workers as even more naturally loving than white women caregivers. In her study, employers consistently thought of their domestic workers as naturally warm, patient, and loving. In other words, the care work of Latina domestic workers is so natural it is effortless. As a consequence, employers negated domestic work and diminished its contribution to economic growth through low wages. Rather than emphasize how domestic work contributes to the economy, employers attributed the labor of domestic workers to their national or ethnic culture.

This ideology that associates women of color with hyperloving care abilities is not new to maintaining economic stratification. Sociologist Bonnie Thornton Dill's classic research on black women's work at the turn of the twentieth century demonstrates that the high proportion of black women in household work was a direct product of slavery.[12] Dominant ideologies justified the presence of black women in slavery by saying that they were both inherently hypersexual and hyperloving. These same ideologies justified job discrimination and poor work conditions for black women post-slavery. Today, white women are the public face of care work and recognized for providing it professionally. In contrast, women of color are concentrated in the "dirty work" of care work, working as maids or kitchen workers.[13] More specifically, Latinas and black women tend to be concentrated in nonnurturing care work, and they are increasingly in lower-paid, nonprofessional nurturing care work.[14] It was at the moment when nursing became professionalized that administrators stopped seeing nurses of color as suitable caregivers.[15] In other words, when care work is legitimized through professionalization it is not as accessible to women of color.

In contrast to women of color, who are idealized as not professional yet naturally hypercaring, male nurses are socially defined as professional and not naturally caring. In contrast to white women who professionally care, male nurses are imagined to be good nurses but primarily in leadership positions.[16] A singular analysis of gender, one that does not consider race, characterizes femininity as naturally meeting the needs of others. In other words, although there are important material distinctions between white women nurses and women of color nurses, it is also important to note a pattern of sameness. To be a woman usually means to provide care in some way or other, and if you are a woman and you do not care, you are a failed woman. By extension, this also means that men do not care naturally and must therefore work very hard to be caring.

In contrast to conventional ideas about the relationship between gender and care, I observed men's abilities and desires to care for patients to be equal to women's. The men in my study said they became nurses because they valued the importance of care and wanted to help people. As Roy, a male charge nurse, explained, "I have no regrets of being a nurse. I get satisfaction out of making people feel better. You know it's rewarding. You know it's always nice when patients come back after having surgery and stuff and say hi and give you a card, a thank-you card. It kind of makes you feel like a hero for that short time, you know. It's kind of neat." Including Roy, nine of the ten male nurses in my study chose nursing because they wanted to be in a helping profession. The remaining nurse said that he later realized that in addition to offering good pay and hours, nursing left him feeling personally satisfied because his work made a difference in people's lives. Male nurses chose to nurse because they enjoyed the caring components of their work and they also wanted to care well. Although drawn from a small sample of only ten male nurses, most of them white, this clear pattern suggests that the feeling of being called to care is not exclusive to women.[17]

Male nurses not only enjoyed the caring components of their work; they also wanted to do it well. They were conscientious about care, often anticipating needs before patients and family members asked. For example, one evening an elderly woman patient in Tom's care expressed a fear of needles and "getting stuck by more people." She was slightly disoriented and anxious. To prevent additional stress, Tom asked a lab technician to check with the unit secretary to see if there were additional orders for blood work before he drew blood from his patient. This way, Tom told me, his patient was stuck only once. In another example, a patient care technician alerted Tom that an elderly female patient's oxygen level was low. When the technician left to get a machine to assist with breathing, Tom calmly observed the patient. He noticed that her demeanor was calm. He considered her negative MRI and angiogram results. After a minute, Tom simply moved the tube from the patient's nose to her mouth. The patient's oxygen level returned to normal. "She is a mouth breather," Tom told me as he ordered a mask to cover her entire face. I observed male nurses like Tom providing gentle, thoughtful care to patients and families on a regular basis. They demonstrated concern through kind words and compassionate facial expressions. Like their women colleagues and contrary to stereotypes about masculinity, male nurses were at ease in handling physically and emotionally intimate or potentially intimate encounters such as rubbing lotion on patients' bodies, holding family members while they grieved, and patiently listening to descriptions of things such as bowel movements.

That men felt called to care and cared well challenges the idea that being caring is a natural attribute of women. Moreover, a closer look at the "ease" with which men provided intimate care revealed how men felt pressure to negotiate the very prevalent idea that they cannot give care. Recall Roy, who said he had "no regrets" about being a nurse. Roy had to articulate his lack of regret because we do not expect masculine people to like nursing. In our interview, he seemed to expect that I would ask if he felt regret, although I did not ask this. His preemptive assertion of "no regret" provides evidence for the dominant ideologies that men do not like to care and do not have the natural ability to care. If we did not question the idea of men in nursing, Roy (and other male nurses) would not mention the possibility of regrets. In order to counteract the idea that they cannot be nurses, men had to figure out how to be feminine and fight against common beliefs about masculinity.

At the same time that Roy said he liked nursing, he used language that suggested he needed to perform "true" masculinity to experience satisfaction as a nurse.[18] For example, he derived his satisfaction at least in part from "feeling like a hero." The relationship between heroism and masculinity is rooted in a strong Western history of what it means to be a man.[19] Scholars who study masculinity in sociology and related fields distinguish men from masculine traits and behaviors. By showing that men (and women) perform masculinity in social interaction, these scholars challenge popular ideas about men, such as the idea that men are naturally aggressive, unemotional, or interested only in heterosexual sex.[20] Masculinity is not a fixed, singular phenomenon and is not something that is naturally linked to men. Women can be masculine, dress masculinely, and act in masculine ways. In addition to showing that masculinity is not biological, gender studies scholars show that masculinities are plural, fluid, shifting, and affected by social power that comes from multiple identities. This scholarship contradicts the notion that masculine traits are inherent to men and shows how naturalizing masculinity to men also supports the idea that femininity is natural to women.

Male nurses described to me how they experienced the effects of dominant images of heterosexual masculinity as unemotional, thoughtless, insensitive, aggressive, dangerous, and violent (especially in intimate situations) in their intimate care work. Many male nurses practiced various forms of mostly mainstream heterosexual masculinity, which drew on ideologies that "true" men were married to women, protected women and children, and possessed physical strength. I also saw men alter conventional ideas of masculinity when they practiced intimate care, because masculine intimacy—especially in professional settings—is often socially coded as violent, aggressive, or sexually inappropriate.[21] For example, men worried that if they showed too much intimacy in their care work, patients—especially women patients—would misinterpret the care male nurses provided them as sexual overtures. When bodily contact was necessary, male nurses discussed how they felt a greater imperative to be more sensitive and cautious than women nurses. They used quick and precise movements because slow movements might have been perceived as lingering and sexually inappropriate.

Brett explained how constructions of masculinity might interfere with his intimate care.

He said, "There is an intimate relationship when you're caring for a patient. When I say that, I mean that there's a sense of compassion and trust. But if you feel disconnected from patients, then you'll be providing care that's not really—not necessarily bad but not necessarily the best, maybe more mediocre." Despite their skills and professional demeanor, male nurses feared that patients and family members could misunderstand their efforts at professional intimacy. Tom explained, "It's harder for males because, [in] this day and age, people [fear] touching other people inappropriately. Oh, I wear gloves all the time. You have to kind of be sterile and let them know that it's a procedure." Roy echoed Tom's sentiments to explain his fears that women patients would misread his professional intimacy as inappropriate behavior:

> It's scary. It's scary being a man. I don't know how the women feel, but it is scary being a man in this field because, you know, being with female patients and stuff. You know, being alone in the room, it is kind of freaky. I know a [male] nurse, just recently, had a complaint. A lady patient came into the ER, and she was, like, totally drunk, and they had to restrain her. And she complained that the charge nurse touched her inappropriately and stuff like that. You know, it's like, geez, you know, anything like that could happen.

Because of masculine and feminine stereotypes involving care, nurturing, touch, and intimacy, male nurses sometimes chose to compromise professional intimacy and err on the side of providing standard care, or what I call *sterile care*. This solved the problem in the short run and may have prevented uncomfortable feelings, but the professional distance resulting from sterile care did not afford the same benefits as professional intimacy.

Sometimes male nurses used traditional ideologies about the institution of marriage to negate any perceived threats or discomfort that might be associated with masculinity. I first observed and interviewed Bill, a white forty-something heterosexual nurse, in the oncology unit. While having her bedpan changed, Bill's patient sarcastically remarked that he would be disgusted by the sight of her exposed body. Bill tried to dilute the comment and redirect the patient's focus from the way she perceived his looking at her by saying, "I'm married." Bill told me that he hoped that his patient would know he was not looking at her sexually and invoked his marital status because he knew it would increase her comfort. It worked. The patient laughed dryly and joked, "You'll never have sex with your wife again!" Here, Bill practiced his "true," heterosexual masculinity specifically in response to how his patient had expressed her insecurities. Since she spoke to him as someone who could be sexually attracted to her, Bill manipulated his masculine gender practice to appear "heterosexual, but uninterested" to ease the discomfort of his patient. He nuanced what is typically considered mainstream hegemonic masculinity by invoking the symbolic meaning of heterosexual marriage: it marked him as stable, unavailable, and sexually appropriate. Bill purposefully disclosed his marital status to his patient because he hoped that this would eliminate her possible discomfort with his need to be intimate with her as part of his work. Bill's negotiation of masculine intimacy both proves Raewyn Connell's theory of multiple masculinities and nuances it: here masculine gender as a social construct is defined through its intersection with beliefs about heterosexuality.[22] Bill's choice to invoke marriage while providing intimate care also serves a foundation for beginning to think of professional intimacy as purposeful labor, not work that accidentally happens because a nurse is inherently nice and compassionate.

It is well documented that male nurses experience patients who perceive them as gay or "too" feminine. The common stereotype that male nurses must be gay should be analyzed at the intersection of feminine gender and gay sexuality. When patients do not assume masculine intimacy is a threat, they assume it is "abnormally" feminine—in other words, gay. Regardless of one's sexual orientation, feminine behavior from men is often perceived by others as gay.[23] Nick, a new nurse, confirmed that patients think male nurses are gay. He said, "And I get that, too. That's another misconception, actually. People, they think males that come into the nursing profession are gay." All male nurses I interviewed commented on the regularity with which their sexual orientation was questioned—both overtly and covertly. This was often done covertly by patients and their families who inquired about a male nurse's marital status and children.

Male nurses experienced questions about their sexual orientation from colleagues, too. Brett explained how other nurses asked similar questions about his sexuality: "Yes, I think they [other nurses] do in a very subtle way. They'll start kind of pulling information from me. 'Are you married? Do you have a girlfriend? Any kids?' And when I first started here, nurses had assigned someone to try to kind of pull some information from me." Some male nurses responded to gay or feminine perceptions about them by asserting they were married. They did this to build trust with their patients because they assumed it would increase their patients' comfort levels. Of course, these nurses had a patient in mind when they made this decision: heterosexual and homophobic. On the other hand, other male nurses practiced femininity on purpose to help women patients feel more comfortable with them. For example, when giving patients baths, Jared took great care in acting what he called "neutral," which was arguably a less aggressive masculinity or perhaps a more feminine masculinity. Jared avoided gruff language and vocal tones. While his voice was not effeminate, it was soft—softer than when he spoke in the nurses' station or when I interviewed him. Jason "played up his feminine side" with patients he knew or assumed to be gay. He purposefully acted more effeminate. At the same time, while Bill sometimes evoked his heterosexual masculinity, I also observed him, as he described it, "play up his feminine side" with men patients he knew or assumed to be gay. He purposefully acted more effeminate with these patients, he said, in case they would be more comfortable thinking he too was gay. Bill told me that *he* was comfortable knowing that his gay patients might assume he also was gay, and patient comfort was his primary goal.

Male nurses were in a bind. They worked hard to disentangle the ways that others conflated gender with sexuality in the process of care. They worked differently—some argue harder—to prove they were caring and intimate in a way that was not sexualized, gay or straight. Male nurses demonstrated that care that is coded masculine could be safe, but only when provided in a way that cannot be perceived as cold or sexual. They needed to be hypercaring—yet hyperprofessional—in their intimacy.

The relationship between intimacy and gender in my study both confirms and disputes conventional ideas of care, masculinity, and femininity. This shows that social ideologies and practices of gender affect the experiences of work for nurses and change the meanings of care, masculinity, and femininity; however, a closer look at what it meant to care revealed that men and women nurses negotiated intimacy differently with their patients by observing, interpreting, and responding to their patients' needs differently. Again, this means that although my observations of male nurses challenged the idea that femininity is an inherent predictor of care, it also confirmed the power and presence of conventional definitions of masculinity and femininity in nursing.

Traditionally, nursing has been considered women's work.[24] Historically, sociologists and other scholars use the phrase *women's work* to indicate how jobs that employ primarily women are also jobs that do not pay well and have less room for advancement when compared to jobs that are historically held by men. The phrase *women's work* consists of care and service tasks that are in keeping with what are considered to be natural attributes held by women. Feminist economists have argued that part of the reason women's work does not pay well is that it emphasizes tasks women "should" do naturally. I see this gendering of nursing play out in recruitment advertisements, which suggest that women (and here women of color) are "born to care." Advertisements for men do not mention care and instead evoke normative ideas of "true" men.[25] From these advertisements, it would seem that men would be interested in nursing because it is a profession that demands strength, but women are interested because it lets them be caring. These ads reinforce the binary that women, not men, are interested in caring and that men have to prove that they would be good nurses.

The phrase *women's work* draws attention to the tensions in nursing that accompany a predominately female labor force. But because men increasingly are nurses, it is useful to distinguish "women's work," which is typically occupied by women, from "feminine work," or work that is gendered as feminine.[26] The phrase *feminine work* draws attention to how gender operates as a social construct in nursing because it makes the distinction between women as bodies and tasks that are typically associated with women's bodies. People and institutions mask the actual labor of traditionally feminine tasks—tasks such as nurturing, serving, and cleaning bodies of other people—because conventional ideas of femininity do not consider care to be "real work" for women but, rather, tasks that "true" women would do naturally.[27]

The idea that true women are naturally caring makes feminine work invisible because there is no need to count what comes naturally, and therefore easily, as labor.[28] These beliefs about women negate the skills necessary for feminine work.[29] Feminine work, especially when conducted by women, is not formally counted as part of professional labor, is taken for granted by employers and employees, and is typically unpaid.

The idea that giving care is a natural trait specific to women is steeped in ideas that equate women's inherent caregiving abilities with women's role in carrying and delivering babies. The relationship between women's reproductive abilities and care is, of course, a belief and not a fact. Although men do not get pregnant, some women also cannot or will not biologically bear children; yet their inability to give birth does not exclude them from this assumption of inherent caregiving abilities. It is not really that women have children so they are naturally caring, it is that women disproportionately raise children that make this idea seem true. Because women traditionally provide the bulk of care work in and outside of the home, it is easier to say that women do women's work more easily than men, even though we all know women who do not seem nurturing and men who seem to nurture with ease.[30]

How we naturalize care as a trait of ideal femininity might explain why new women nurses feel pressured to inherently know how to provide intimate care for patients and why new male nurses feel out of their element. The nurse directors in my study explained care by drawing on traditional ideas of femininity—in this case, how women are primarily responsible for child care. Anita, a nurse director introduced in the Introduction, described how her skills as a mother served her as a nurse: "I have four children. So did having children prepare me? I mean, I was a nurse first, but did having four children and multiple demands teach me how to handle multiple patients or a unit with different personalities? Or did my education help me with my family? I don't know what came first, but I think I'm good at both of them. They do take some of the same skills." Other nurse directors encouraged their staff nurses to nurture their patients as they would family members. To new nurses, Peggy, a nurse director, recommends, "Try to treat your patients like a loved one, somebody they love, whoever means the most to you, whoever they cherish." Molly also "make[s her] nurses understand the importance of care" by telling them, "Would you like your mother taken care of in this situation by you?" These directors' analyses of care highlight the relationship between being a caring nurse and traditional expectations of femininity, such as motherhood and nurturing family members. This relationship keeps the labor of care a mystery and sustains the idea that women should be naturally caring.

Many practitioners think that if nurses cannot intuitively care for patients, they should not be nurses.[31] Through their expectations of job performance, nurse directors reinforced the relationships among femininity, care, and nursing. Some administrators, like Anita, assumed that nurses are naturally caring: "Nurses are usually pretty caring and by nature do not deal well with conflict. They kind of stuff it. They don't like confrontation." Peggy also believed that "everyone enters the profession because they have a true caring and compassion for people" and that "nursing is one those fields which attracts women." Other directors, like Molly, emphasized technical skill but then clearly stated they want nurses to show compassion for patients. She told me, "My expectations are for nurses to be technically good, but it goes beyond technical. I expect them to be professional and to provide caring, compassion—to also be compassionate to the patient." These assertions suggest that caring is either an innate trait or an emotional state that nurses should easily possess by sympathizing with their patients.

Nurse directors emphasized the relationships among care, instinct, and femininity by discussing care as a unique trait. Anita described a nurse who is very good at caring: "I think it has to do with her own personal energy. I think she naturally delivers care in a way that is loving, comforting, more physical. Another nurse might do it differently." Molly assessed a new nurse by her "positive energy," too:

She's very pretty and just had a sparkly personality, and all the patients just loved her. Technically, she was a very mediocre nurse, but everyone just loved her because she was pretty and sparkly, and I loved her, too—she was a lot younger—like a big sister. She was a wonderful person, and she's an example of how she looked and how she was; she was real sweet. They [the patients] thought they were getting the best care and sang her praises. I would want more technically experienced nurses taking care of me; there is a difference between technical nursing and the caring.

In her description of this nurse, Molly separates technical skill from caring ability. Moreover, she focused on this nurse's individual personality traits. The patients loved Molly's nurse because she was "sparkly" and "sweet." Molly drew on traditional notions of femininity as pleasing others to define care. Although they may not have meant to, because it risks the professionalism of nursing, nurse directors explicitly related being naturally sweet and charismatic to caring well for patients. When Anita emphasized that other nurses could care as well as the nurse she described, but do so differently, she contributed to the erasure of skill and work in caring because she identified care as an individual personality trait. Nurses did skillfully negotiate intimacy, but describing care as a unique personality trait makes it difficult to pinpoint patterns, which would help articulate care as a skill that can be taught.

The myth of Florence Nightingale persists today; it informs how patients, administrators, and the general public naturalize care.[32] Defining good nurses as "nightingales" and "angels of mercy" mystifies care as a personal attribute rather than something that can be learned over time. My field notes show that even nurses understood their skilled care work as something that "just naturally happens over time" rather than as a product of training. For example, many nurses could not say exactly how they cared for patients, saying instead, "I don't know" or "I just do it." When I asked how they learned to do specific tasks or handle intimate situations, nurses said they learned from experience or from other nurses. Nurses also used personal characteristics, rather than labor activities, to differentiate nursing in different units of the hospital. For example, they described themselves and others who work in oncology as "kind," "soft," and "patient," nurses in intensive care as "quick-thinking" and "intelligent," and nurses in the ER as "tough" and "able to handle anything." When nurses use personality characteristics to describe their labor, it makes it harder to recognize it as work that is indispensable to health, well-being, and saving lives.

Care as a natural feminine trait contributes to the fantasy of care. Patients described "good" nurses as those who provide care that results in good interactions. Through experience, nurses learned when to emphasize the positive and minimize the negative in their caregiving efforts. Over time, this know-how looked natural, and administrators and educators defined it as a personality characteristic. Nurses, patients, and others described good care as something that happens naturally in part because there was no professional language to describe how nurses negotiate intimacy in care. Moreover, this appearance of naturalness sustained the idea that quality health care is inherently defined through goodness. When conflict happened, nurses were worried that administrators would hold them accountable and say they were not doing their job.

We can challenge these ideas by showing how they are rooted in historical and contemporary ideologies of nursing, women, and femininity, which do more than naturalize care to women. They exclude men and pressure new women nurses to possess natural caregiving abilities in the workplace. The association between naturalness and care also glorifies care as something that nurses do well and not something for which they are professionally trained. Naturalizing care—that is, assuming that individuals are naturally caring— can help simplify nurses' work from the perspective of patients who are overrun and overwhelmed by their illnesses and do not want to worry about *how* their nurses care but just want to know that they do. While perhaps helpful to patients, naturalizing care also obscures how nurses negotiate intimacy and conflict with and among patients and family members.

Moralizing Nurses, Moralizing Nursing

There is a relationship between moralizing and naturalizing care. Naturalizing care suggests that nurses—women in particular—are naturally good at caring and do not have to work at it. Moralizing care is what "good," "natural" caregivers do. They provide care as a gift that is given to patients and do not need professional expertise that requires training and practice. Using rhetoric that suggests care work is a gift, a calling, or a sacrifice fails to acknowledge the intimate labor of care. Instead, this rhetoric glorifies care as a universal gift given by nurses or as an all-encompassing moral ethic that all good people should adopt.

Alongside the myth that care is an inherent personality trait in women runs a deeply rooted philosophy that prioritizes compassion for patients as a moral duty. Many of the nurses I studied told me they entered nursing because they wanted to honor and heal the sick and care for the ill and injured. Even nurses who did not enter nursing for these reasons found patient care to be one of the most satisfying aspects of their work because they felt that it gave them the opportunity to act out their moral principles. This is not a new idea. Nursing was founded in part on the principle that care is a feminine virtue and a way for women to act on their moral beliefs.[33] Today, nurses around the world emphasize the moral and spiritual aspects of care to demonstrate how care improves social life in general. They do this in part to increase social value of their labor; however, doing so also detracts from economics and other work conditions.

Part of the problem is that when nurses define care, they are not talking about care as intimate work. Rather, they talk about care as a value. Separate from the professional recognition of nursing runs a deeply instilled philosophy that prioritizes compassion for patients above all other tasks. The ideology of care operates as the conscience of nursing, with values that include providing faith and hope; sensitivity to self and others; and a supportive, protective, and healing environment. Nurses tend to value care as a foundational premise in nursing, yet few recognize it as professional labor.

Almost from the beginning of my study, I observed the relationship between the talk of intimacy and the assessment of nurses' care work. I began to see how nurses and administrators defined "good" nurses as naturally and morally caring and "bad" nurses as those who struggled with being caring or did not always feel the call. In fact, many of the senior nurses and the nursing administrators talked about a generational divide in nursing: that new nurses are not as motivated to care as the senior nurses and administrators and are in nursing for only the money. Other administrators explained how new nurses seemed less adept at caring for patients by suggesting they must be in the job for the money, not for the patients. This explanation (that new nurses were in it for the money and not for the patients) supports the ideas that care is natural and that only naturally caring individuals have the moral desire to nurse and nonnaturally caring individuals do not have the ability to nurse since the ability to care is not a learned trait. It also suggests that money is not always a part of nursing and that nurses are incompetent if they care about their salaries. This reinforces the idea that nursing is really a calling and not a job and challenges its status as a profession. Instead of acknowledging that money affects motivations for most jobs, nurse administrators and some experienced bedside nurses demonized new nurses by suggesting they spoil the profession.

The money or care sentiment is another false binary that affected how administrators assessed the competency of nurses. Good nurses did not talk about money; bad nurses cared about only money. Good nurses are natural caregivers who feel mercy for the sick. Good nurses sacrifice themselves for their patients. They feel a sense of moral obligation to healing that supersedes compensation. Good nurses create care through their natural abilities or through their moral ethics. These strict and false relationships between good nurses and mercy, good nurses and sacrifice, good nurses and duty begin—at least in our social imagination—in the actual material conditions of some of the first nurses, nursing nuns.[34]

It is important to understand the idea of care as moral duty within the social and economic history of nursing. By draping the profession of nursing in the "true womanhood" ideals of purity, piety, domesticity, and submissiveness, nurses were better protected from sexual objectification and social disgrace. This was especially important as the medical industry modernized and increasingly placed nurses in submissive positions under doctors. As a result of this subordination and the disorderly conditions of hospitals during this time, moral reformers like Florence Nightingale advocated for nurses' independent working conditions by reverting back to these ideals of true womanhood. This helped them gain and maintain respect.[35]

Today, this ideology of care as a moral ethic operates as the conscience of nursing, with values that include provision of faith and hope; sensitivity to self and others; and a supportive, protective, and healing environment. Renowned nursing theorist Jean Watson defines care as a sacred science that considers a deeper ethical belief system having worldwide implications for a more just, peaceful society.[36] Nurses and the general public describe nursing as sacred work—work that is quasi-religious and rich with ritual.[37] These images implicate nurses in their daily practice, making them responsible not just for care of their patients but also for world peace.[38] The good nurse is an angel, the nurse who is naturally called to nursing, rather than the nurse who provides good care because of her training and expertise.[39]

Professionalizing Nursing

I discovered that administrative nurses did not talk about intimacy because they were concerned that doing so would degrade their profession by invoking the fantasy of the "sexy nurse." Nurses would then not be taken seriously as professional workers. This is a valid concern. Historically, people have viewed nurses as maternal figures, angels of mercy, or seductive temptresses.[40] In response, nurses have struggled to define their labor so that it is duly recognized as work that is indispensable to health, well-being, and saving lives.

Professionalization has been one way that nurses have promoted the skill and complexity of their labor. Nursing used to be considered "sacred" work, "a calling" for white middle-class women, or the only job accessible to women other than teaching; now it is a career path viewed as suitable for men and women of various races, classes, and ethnicities. One need only visit the Internet website of the American Nurses Association or peruse the shelves in any university health sciences library to see concrete evidence of the professionalization of nursing. Nurses conceptualize, develop, test, and practice medical and, increasingly, technical knowledge. They create and maintain sustainable venues for research, publication, and teaching in academic degree programs. The nursing profession maintains ethical and best-practices standards for education and research, illness assessment and diagnosis practices, delegation of roles and responsibilities, and documentation.

To maintain their professional image, I found, nurse administrators in my study created a false division between professionalism and intimacy. By this I mean that administrators decisively said that nurses who were professional could not be intimate with their patients and nurses who were intimate had trouble being professional; that is, intimate nurses lacked the ability to demonstrate and assess specialized medical and technical information. This falsity rests on the artificial belief that to be caring is something one does naturally, through intuition, or as a moral activity. At the same time that administrators maintained that intimacy was not part of nursing, they quickly pointed out that nurses had to be caring, too. Nurse administrators expected nurses to be naturally caring and were surprised when they were not.

Experienced nurses knew that part of their job was to make the hard work of negotiating intimacy look easy because it made patients feel more comfortable but that to talk about intimacy would detract from their professional authority. Many nurses I spoke with could not or would not always articulate the process of intimacy in care. They insisted that nursing did not involve intimacy—which was often conflated with sexuality—and to say that it did would minimize the professionalism of their work. Although nurses strive for professional recognition of their labor, administrators and the general public discuss care labor without specifying the skill and specialized knowledge necessary for intimate encounters with patients and family members. According to the nurse directors I interviewed, nursing straddles a dichotomy where the nurse is either nurturing or rational, neither of which addresses intimate labor. When the nurse is discussed as nurturing, administrators describe nursing care as natural and virtuous traits inherent to certain individuals. When the nurse is discussed as rational, administrators explain nursing care as a set of medical or technical skills that can be taught. This false binary between virtue and skill precludes an assessment of how the two function simultaneously in nursing.

Although nurses rarely acknowledged that they did so, I observed how they combined gentleness and shrewdness to respond to the changing needs of patients and family members and the schedules and resources of other clinical staff. Nurses made decisions in fast-paced and rapidly shifting environments. They were as skillful in their medical knowledge and decision making as they were in managing emotions and drying tears. To say that nursing is either intimate or intellectual loses sight of the work conditions that nurses must face every day[41] and does not prepare new nurses for work that combines both aspects.[42] Nonetheless, most nurses discuss the value of intimate care, but few recognize care as conflict negotiation that requires professional knowledge, skill, and practice.

A perhaps unintended consequence of separating intimacy from professionalism was that it diluted the importance of care. At the same time, nurses—especially bedside nurses—struggled with articulating the importance of care in nursing. This is more the case now that medical practice and hospital stays seem to be driven by health management organizations rather than the needs of patients.[43] The bedside nurses in my study felt torn and suffered what feminist philosopher Marilyn Frye called a double bind.[44] If nurses focus their attention and time on patient care, they fail to be efficient. If they focus on cost, they fail to care. In both cases they fail, and it is a "lose-lose" situation. This institutional condition causes nurses to experience additional stress in an already burdensome workday. Let me offer an example from my notes at the beginning of my study:

> I am having informal conversations with nursing educators and clinicians across the United States, from New York City to Portland and from Boise to Phoenix. In these conversations, I hear nurses (sometimes in the same conversation) explain care as professional work that requires training and as a personality trait some nurses naturally possess and as skilled labor. On the one hand, nurses know that their work in general is professional. On the other, they insist that women are "naturally more caring than men." At first, these claims seem contradictory; how can nurses say both that their labor is professional and that it is not? The answer is in how nurses do not specifically delineate care apart from other tasks. They are very clear about how they are professional but seem to take care for granted. It is as if they cannot acknowledge their own work that makes the experience of feeling care natural to the patient.[45]

I interpreted nurses saying that care was professional as indicative of how established ways of talking about professional work do not allow space for emotions or intimacy. Traditional definitions of professionalism suggest that to be professional, one should remain objective and emotionally neutral in the workplace. This is a dilemma for any professionals who must negotiate emotion as part of their work. In part, nurses emphasize professionalism in their labor so that their labor will be taken seriously as a health science, but professionalism in nursing creates a false binary.[46] False binaries frame an aspect of society in opposites: black or white, girl or boy, professional or emotional. False binaries are false because the binary of either/or does not capture the whole complexity of the experience. Nurses are caught in another double bind. On the one hand, intimacy detracts from professionalization. On the other hand, negotiating intimacy is part of care work in nursing. Nurses, then, are in the tricky spot of making their intimate labor appear to not be work to make patients feel comfortable and also to make nurses appear more professional. A focus on professionalization erases the work of intimate care. When nurses erase intimacy from their work, it leaves little room to articulate how intimacy is negotiated and the harm they could experience when negotiating this intimacy.

Nurses who make negotiating intimate care seem natural for their patients also may minimize harm when it happens as part of intimate care exchanges. The new nurses I studied were not prepared to consider how intimate care may make their patients feel sexually entitled to them and display inappropriate sexual behaviors. Although nurses generally feel uneasy about discussing sexuality as part of their work, some nursing scholars recognize how sexuality affects the nurse-patient relationship and have advocated for including sexuality in nursing education.[47]

Throughout my study, I learned that nurses very seriously and regularly negotiated the sexuality of patients and sexual attention from patients. In a medical-surgical unit, for example, I observed several nurses "handle" a patient who consistently masturbated in bed. Nurses also negotiated sexual relations between patients and visitors, especially during nighttime hours. Moreover, nurses consistently managed comments and touches from patients. Studies of sexual harassment in nursing confirm that the most common perpetrators are patients,[48] although most employment policies and trade journals focus on how physicians and administrators sexually harass nurses.[49] These studies describe how nurses feel shame and humiliation when dealing with harassing and abusive patients, which disrupts the quality of health care.[50]

Based on these studies, I first thought that I would study sexual harassment from patients in nursing. When I began the study, I met with unit directors to help me recruit participants. When I mentioned (quite seriously) that I wanted to discern harmful intimacies that cause and result from conflict, such as sexual harassment, from intimacies that were helpful and necessary for care work, nurse directors laughed at me and rolled their eyes. Immediately, one of the directors burst out with, "What? You can't talk about *sex* and *intimacy* with nurses. They'll laugh you out of the room." Other unit directors smiled and nodded their heads in agreement. I clearly had a lot to learn. When I met with each of the unit directors individually, each gently suggested that I avoid using words like *sexual*, even when asking about sexual harassment in my formal interviews, project description, and informal conversations. They worried—perhaps rightly so—that nurses would not take me seriously.[51]

Other administrators were confused about my focus on inappropriate sexual behaviors from patients. When I met with the director of human resources, she told me that nurses did not report sexual harassment from patients. All administrators agreed that some patients displayed inappropriate sexual desire to nurses but that good nurses adeptly managed their interactions with patients. They said that professional nurses controlled patients, not the other way around. According to these directors, when nurses have authority over their patients, they do not experience sexual harassment or other kinds of intimate conflicts from patients.

Here, we see not only that professionalism requires nurses to minimize the reality of intimacy and sexuality in their work but also that nurses draw on the rhetoric of professionalism to explain how they address harm or conflict that results from intimacy. Bedside nurses experience yet another double bind. Professional nurses should be able to handle sexual indiscretions or other negative intimacies from their patients; however, handling intimacy is not a part of formal training. Throughout my observations, I witnessed experienced nurses easily negotiate harmful intimacies, but new nurses were lost. New nurses were baffled when patients interacted with them on any sexual level. While perhaps they experienced sexual harassment from their colleagues or their supervisors, they told me they would have never expected it from patients. When I asked new nurses why they felt this way, they overwhelmingly described how they viewed patients as needy and dependent. In other words, they were not used to seeing people they were hired to help as potentially harmful.

The possibility of a patient being a harasser significantly disrupts normative definitions of harassers. By this I mean that when we normally think of harassers we likely draw on popular policy, news, and legal rhetoric and images that describe harassers as people with power who use this power to get what they want. Moreover, we tend to think of potential harassment as something that happens at work, coming from bosses or colleagues, or in public, coming from strangers. We likely think of bosses or colleagues first, and then we might consider the kind of harassment that occurs from someone we do not know, on the street or at a party. We think of harassers as active, controlling, and powerful. We rarely, if ever, think of harassers who are ill or in any other way dependent.

Feminist philosophers Eva Feder Kittay and Ellen Feder[52] challenge the false binary of independence and dependence, especially as it relates to one's agency or having control over oneself. Typically, we associate agency with independence. The relationship between independence and agency masks how definitions of independence actually rely on the existence of dependence. Consider the statement "I know I am independent when I am not dependent." Sometimes, when meanings of agency are conflated with meanings of independence, this statement becomes, "I know I have agency when I am independent, and therefore I cannot have control over my own actions when I am dependent." In my research I consistently found that nurses describe patients by talking about their neediness, dependence, and, therefore, their inability to intend harm from their actions. In my first study on nursing, nurses described that they negotiated patients' sexuality as part of their job, but did not feel harmed.[53] Although nurses discussed unwelcome and persistent sexual behaviors from patients, they did not define these as sexual harassment. Nurses strategically avoided labeling their interactions with patients in a way that would potentially criminalize those who needed their care. Instead, they justified patients' sexual and violent behaviors toward them, claiming that these individuals were merely "patients who were confused" or saying that "it is part of their [the patients'] illness."

To maintain naturalized ideas about care (that it is good and pure and not spoiled by harm), nurses could not talk about sexuality in any forms ranging from positive intimacy to sexual harassment. Moreover, to discuss sexuality would detract from the professionalism of nursing. Talking about sexuality would also detract from the idea that patients are needy, dependent, and grateful. How nurses negotiate trust and conflict in intimate care labor remains in large part unnamed in nursing. Instead, educators and employers encourage nurses to imagine patients who provoke them as inherently good in order to care for them.[54] This portrayal of patients makes invisible how nurses manage positive and negative intimacy as part of care. As nurse director Molly said to me:

> When nurses get into nursing, they have no idea the intimacy you get involved with until you're out of school. I mean, while you are in school, you're not thinking about that, but when you get out there and get your job, and you're like, is this all there is? Is this what it is? And you realize, oh gosh, you have to spend time intimately close with a lot of people who are not happy and sick. It's draining, and if you are a person who isn't real solid and who gets stressed and can't handle a lot of the emotional stuff, it's hard.

I quickly discovered that intimacy, not sexual harassment, was the elephant in the room with nurses. People knew about intimacy but worked hard to ignore it or deny its existence. It was then that I realized (partly in retrospect) I had heard no talk of intimacy in general conversation or as part of medical practice. As mentioned previously, when I asked directly about intimacy in care work, many new nurses denied its presence entirely or acted as if intimacy did not include conflict. Conversely, several directors admitted that new nurses were not prepared to handle intimacy or the conflict that comes from intimacy.

Bedside Care as Skilled Work

To address these images of nursing as a calling and nurses as angels of mercy, nurses use professionalism to increase visibility and add value to their skills, knowledge, and contributions to the medical profession; however, emphasizing professionalism minimizes the importance of care, especially when compared to science and technology. Moreover, this emphasis further takes caring abilities for granted. As the value of professionalism increased in the nursing industry, some nursing scholars worried that the value of bedside care was decreasing. One nursing scholar in particular rose to the top with her theories of care as skilled labor. Since 1984, Patricia Benner's model of expert nursing has continued to inspire and shape bedside nursing practices from the perspectives of bedside nurses around the world. Benner defines care as expert skill from the perspective of expert nurses but does not acknowledge the role of institutional social and economic power.

In her landmark work *From Novice to Expert* (1984), Patricia Benner addresses how nurses separate care work from professionalism by showing that care can be measured as skill acquisition rather than as a personality trait or an individual talent. She argues that the nursing industry's focus on standardizing technical skill and medical knowledge misses the most important part of nursing labor—care. Benner contends that the only way nurses can obtain this knowledge is through exemplars from nurses, because experienced nurses teach detailed understandings of caring interactions. She further posits that we must focus on the expertise of nurses to comprehensively learn about the dynamics of care.

Benner's approach defines care as a constructed interaction in which nurses actively involve their patients. In this approach, care occurs in the relationship between the nurse and the patient and cannot be controlled through the kinds of routines or standardization of practices found in typical professional discourse. Benner argues that knowledge about how to care for patients

transcends standardization procedures because it is embedded in individualized clinical practices with patients. She asserts the importance of nurses'
perceptual abilities and how nurses provide comfort and communication
through touch, support to families, and reassuring presence at the bedside,
and by maximizing patients' feelings of control over a situation. According to
Benner's theory, nurses become expert caregivers when they can judge situations, understand the unique conditions of individual patients, and make
exceptions when needed. Benner's model allows new nurses to learn from
expert nurses and advance at work when they demonstrate these specialized
skills. She argues that nurses and hospital administrators can facilitate, recognize, and reward care as professional skill.[55]

Although written in 1984, Benner's work is currently relevant in nursing
education, career development, and training programs.[56] Benner challenges
the nursing industry to consider how nurses should learn thematic aspects
of care rather than procedures and routines. Her work helped the industry
begin to view clinical care as professional practice, and it significantly affects
how nurses think about and provide care today. Benner's model of expert
care now informs certification exams and nursing curriculums in the United
States,[57] Canada, Australia, Great Britain,[58] and Scotland.[59] It also influences
nursing policies and procedures in New Zealand.[60] It informs research studies
on care and a professional work model marketed by Richard Benner (the husband of Patricia Brenner) and his associates to health-care providers.[61] Nurses
continue to recognize how care is restricted by national policies, protocols,
and guidelines.[62] In the 1980s, Patricia Benner's model influenced a renewed
recognition and call for mentorships and preceptors in nursing as a solution
to the nursing shortage by encouraging nurse retention.[63] Benner's work also
challenges the definition of care as natural, especially as it relates to nursing
education and practice.[64]

More than twenty years after Patricia Benner published *From Novice to
Expert*, I find we still need a language to describe the profession of intimate
care in nursing. Although it seeks to contribute to the professionalization of
nursing, Benner's philosophy of nursing care is rooted in the same historical
ideologies of nursing that suggest there is an intrinsic relationship between
moral beliefs about care and moral practices of care.[65] These ideas suggest
that "true" care does not include discomfort or conflict for the nurse. In other
words, "true," "good" nurses do not feel discomfort in the ways they alleviate discomfort for patients. My findings suggest otherwise. Only when we
discuss how care includes conflict can we really begin to envision ways to
encourage hospitals to support these efforts. Benner suggests that it is only
routine that disrupts the interaction of care, but other parties also control

care. Health management organizations control care. Administrators control care. Patients control care. And each of these has vested interests and responsibilities in the care process.

Benner claims that expert knowledge can be facilitated in a hospital setting, but I argue that facilitation can occur only if we accept that there is no one expert way to care. Rather, the expertise of intimate care might be in how nurses professionally negotiate intimacy as a conduit between the medical industry and the patient to ensure that the patient receives quality health care. While Benner argues that care is constructed in interactions and in the context of these interactions, she does not discuss how care is a social event. It is still important to highlight how care is skilled and can be understood by analyzing individual nurses' experiences and meanings of their own work, yet it is critical that we explain how care changes according to social and economic contexts to reflect the structural patterns of nursing.[66]

In contrast to Benner, I do not think the nurse-patient relationship is unique. I think we can learn from nurses to show how care can be negotiated and understood in other social and work contexts. My project is to provide a sociological perspective of intimacy in care as it occurs in nursing and to discuss the management of this intimacy neither as a calling nor as a commitment but as a condition of professional caring labor.

Seeing Intimacy: Intersectionality and Commercialized Intimacy

In spite of the fantasy that intimate care just naturally happens, I watched how experienced nurses consistently coordinated the process of patient care—with doctors, with other hospital departments, with family members, and with the patients themselves. Sitting in the nurses' station, I began to pay attention to how care is a process, how nurses coordinate the care process, and how intimate labor is essential for quality patient care to occur. Had I just stayed in the nurses' station, the only expertise I would have witnessed would have been medical and administrative coordination. It was not until I started following nurses into patient rooms that I saw the difference between intimacy and care. In the oncology unit, I first noticed the connection between how coordinating care is invisible labor and how intimacy in care work went unnoticed by all parties: patients, family members, doctors, hospital administrators, and even nurses. If no one pays attention to how departments, specialists, and other care providers are connected, surely no one will understand the importance of developing and maintaining trust with patients to help ensure quality health care.

In each unit, but beginning in oncology, I began to think about how new nurses are not prepared to manage intimate care but experienced nurses make the process of care appear natural and easy as a way to help reassure patients and family members. I realized that managing intimate care is not part of any discussion about nursing in the hospital where I conducted my study, despite the fact that this hospital is recognized as being in the top 2 percent of this nation's hospitals for quality of nursing care. Because I saw how nurses must document virtually every move they make, I asked administrators how care is also assessed. One administrator, an experienced researcher, laughed and told me that being caring does not get measured. "How could it?" she asked. She—like other nurses and administrators in this hospital—knew that there was a caring quality that needed to be a part of "patient care" but thought that nurses naturally brought caring with them. Over the course of planning and conducting my study, I learned that many nurses think that for a nurse to be a good nurse, she or he must possess the natural ability to care for others. I learned that while some nurses were intrigued with my idea that care could be taught, most nurses insisted otherwise: nurses must be caring, but it is a natural trait. It cannot be charted or assessed, and it certainly cannot be taught.

How did nurses not know that they were teaching the very thing that they said could not be taught? Intimate care work is also invisible, because although "patient care" encompasses four areas—medical expertise, technical knowledge, coordination skill, and intimate interactions—the last aspect, intimacy, is not valued as knowledge or skill. Because care work is an umbrella definition for these four aspects and because intimacy is not marked, a specific aspect of care—negotiating intimacy—gets lost in the discussion. The value of care is hypervisible in this hospital, but the process of care is unrecognized. It was here that I realized that talking about only the value of care and not the process of care contributes to the fantasy of care, which universalizes care as natural and makes intimacy—good and bad—invisible.

Although patient care was compartmentalized in distinct departments (medical care, emotional therapy, physical therapy, social work, housekeeping, dietary, and so on), the nurses I observed and interviewed felt responsible for their patients' entire experience and stay in the hospital. They coordinated the entire process of care. "Total patient care" as the hospital defined it was divided among administrative, service, and care tasks, each of which are the responsibility of various health-care jobs—that is, housekeeping, unit secretary, case manager, and dietitian. Despite the fact that patients relied on and encountered other medical staff, nurses were the point people for care—the ones who will know at any given moment the needs and status of patients. I saw patients, family members, laboratory technicians, respiratory therapists, nurse assistants, charge nurses, and administrators turning first to the patients' nurse to answer immediate questions or address needs.

Because the job "to care about patients" remains undefined, nurses fulfill their feelings of responsibility for care by coordinating the process. I first noticed this pattern in the oncology unit, although I later saw the same dynamics in the rest of the units I studied. As a result, nurses made sure that patients were educated (informed about their illness and progress) and that their ongoing needs were met. The nurses I observed were always ready to answer a question, and rarely did they defer work to someone else. They tidied up the room between housekeeping visits. They answered the phone when patients were elsewhere in the hospital. They grabbed snacks for patients between meals. They acted as counselor, social worker, and friend:

> I watched Helen, an experienced oncology nurse, talking to a patient with AIDS who was nervous about discharge because he would be going home. She approached him and asked him why he was nervous, and he said because he didn't think his mother could take care of him. Helen told him, "You are fighting for your mom and dad, not because you have the fight in you." He broke into tears and said, "You are right. I do not want to do this anymore." Helen said, "I know your family refused hospice, and I don't want to step on any toes, but there are alternative programs with hospice. It doesn't mean 'end of life.'" The patient said he wanted counseling and that he was interested in outreach programs that would involve his family.[67]

Caring is sometimes talking about difficult issues: whether or not to turn to hospice, to resuscitate, or to "let go." Helen told me that it is the nurses who have these difficult conversations when doctors give patients and family members false hope. Helen knew that oncology is considered "soft" nursing, which means a pace and tone of nursing that is slower than and not as chaotic as departments like the emergency room and intensive care. Sometimes, in the informal lexicon of nursing, "soft" nursing is nursing that lets nurses spend more time with patients, but does not provide as much challenge as the other departments. In contrast, Helen told me that soft nursing does not necessarily ensure comfort. Care also includes being the one who provides the realistic prognosis. Helen did not see herself as a "hand-holder." She saw herself as both compassionate and strong.

Having watched this interaction and talked with Helen afterward, I began to understand the distinction between care and intimacy in hospital nursing. Care is an umbrella word for all interactions with patients, but it also delineates specific areas of knowledge: medical, technical, administrative, and intimate. Moreover, while we rightly define care as therapeutic, we wrongly conflate *all* therapeutic interactions with those that are positive, are nice, and result in all parties feeling good about them. The provision of care can be messy; nurses and patients mix emotions, personalities, and bodily fluids. Sometimes intimacy feels routine to nurses, such as when they are emptying a catheter, checking a wound site, or changing a bandage, but it is the intimate aspect of the interaction that can cause conflict, because patients react to their vulnerabilities in various ways. Some patients show appreciation. Some patients get angry and frustrated. Some patients need extraordinary attention. Some patients harass and abuse nurses. Nurses who care well in all these situations do so because they have knowledge about how to negotiate intimacy.

This intimacy between Helen and her patient was invisible to the rest of the hospital. Because she was required to do so in his chart, Helen noted only that her patient wanted hospice referral, not the process of the interaction that facilitated this knowledge. This is not a bad thing. Nurses are overrun with work, and the last thing they need is more required documentation. At the same time, the chart is the only way to really document the labor of nurses. Much of nurses' work remains unnoticed or uncounted. Nurses are responsible for total patient care but do not have the authority to administer or direct these tasks and processes alone. They rely on other staff whose duties are clearly delineated and who can walk away and leave the unit. Nurses take on the accountability for total patient care but do not receive support or reward for these efforts. Charting documents some of care work. The problem here is that nurses sometimes do not have time to chart until much later on in their shift, but patients' statuses change on a moment's notice. Much of this information is stored in a nurse's head as she moves quickly from patient to patient. Even if a chart is up to date, the standardized method rarely includes "subjective" information regarding a patient's demeanor, attitude, and difficulties. This work is considered subjective in part because it is not counted as institutional knowledge. Seeing the work of intimate care will help explicate the meaning of care and will clarify the work that nurses do.

Centering intimacy in the analysis of care work helps us see how intimacy is both important and invisible in the provision of hospital nursing care. Although the medical industry in general gives priority to technical and medical knowledge, this book foregrounds intimacy in nursing care by defining it as a social construct at work. Social constructs help explain everyday life events through how people and groups of people agree to these meanings and definitions. As a social construct, intimacy and care are not natural feelings, states of being, and events; they are created in and through social interaction, groups, practices, ideas, and values. This does not mean that intimacy or care never feel natural; it just means that for the purposes of this analysis, the meaning of intimacy is more than these emotional experiences.

2

Social and Commercial Aspects
of Intimate Care Work

n February, I began observing the largest, most racially and ethnically diverse staffed unit in the hospital, which the director, Mary, jokingly called the United Nations. At any one time, seven nurses and five patient care technicians shared the work of caring for up to thirty-six patients. There were forty nurses in all, of whom four were from the Philippines, two from Ethiopia, one from Bosnia, and one from Congo. When I began observing this unit, I started to fully understand how social constructions of race and nationality informed the meaning and practice of professionally intimate care:

> About sixteen people were crammed into what looked like the staff lounge but was called a conference room. There were lockers; a bathroom; a rectangular table in the center, chairs, and homemade chocolate on the table; a bulletin board with hospital notices; and a place to hang coats, a small loveseat, and a television. At a staff meeting, Leah, one of the charge nurses and a Filipina woman, said that a patient complained to her that there were nurses "of so many colors." This patient specifically wanted a white nurse. This same patient (this week) "fired" a patient care technician for not being white. Essentially, she refused care from her. The unit director is really amazed that this happens but sees it happening more frequently.[1]

All nurses talked about how these "firings" disrupted how nurses managed the process of care in the unit. As is discussed later in this book, nurses from all racial backgrounds agreed that some white patients expressed their fears and anxieties about their illness through racist attitudes, behaviors, and harassment. These interactions were shaped specifically at various intersections of race, gender, and nationality. Many white nurses along with many women of color nurses agreed that seemingly neutral complaints—complaints that do not mention race, nationality, or citizenship—about nurses of color were likely rooted in distrust because of racist and xenophobic attitudes. Nurses of color feared that these interactions could warp how managers perceive their abilities and could negatively affect assessments of their work.

In this chapter, I introduce how intimate care work is social and economic in nature.[2] I extend this analysis using the intersectional approach to serve as a foundation for professional intimacy. When analyzed by gender, nurses are socially and economically devalued in professional care work because they have been undervalued in a medical industry dominated by men.[3] Nursing has also been devalued in part because it is considered women's work, which is not "real labor" for women but, rather, tasks that all "true" women do naturally.[4] Although they have been useful for revealing the gendered dynamic in hospitals, the studies I cite in the preceding two sentences are problematic because they center gender as the explanatory factor and universalize white English-speaking women's experiences as all women's experiences. Sociological and feminist theories teach us that explaining the effect of multiple identities is crucial to understanding experience.

Just as emotions might feel natural to us, so could our gender, race, sexuality, and nationality identities. This means that many of us think that our identities are a personal part of us and do not affect the way we experience the world in any political way. We tend to think of our identities as personal and believe that they do not affect whether or not we have opportunities or disadvantages. Although we may experience gender, race, sexuality, and nationality as personal identities, sociologists define identities as social categories that are shaped by social ideologies, institutions, and interactions. This means that whether or not we pay attention to them, our identities shape our experiences in the world, including how we access opportunities and resources as well as how we experience oppression and discrimination. Naming social identities—social constructs—does two things: first, it distinguishes talking about identity in a social way from how identity is personally experienced; and second, it indicates that as members of society, individuals and groups participate in constructing the meaning of social identities.

If we say that people agree to meanings of social constructs—both events and identities—we can also argue that they disagree. The meanings of these categories are not fixed, because they are based on the perceptions and experiences of individuals and groups. Social practices and ideas change over time, and these changes affect how meanings of social ideas, practices, and events change. In other words, sometimes you know that a social, cultural, political, or economic idea is socially constructed by how it changes over time and by geographic region. Sociologists study personal identities as social constructs to help explain how societal views on race, gender, sexuality, and nationality change over time and according to where we live.

Members of society continuously socially construct the meanings of identities by creating a relationship between identity and specific values and beliefs. People reinforce these meanings by practicing them in social interactions and regulating them through social institutions. In other words, we create social constructs; we express and perform them, we perceive them, and we identify with them. Over time and reinforced through various elements of society, people experience socially constructed identities as natural and normal. This makes the meanings of social constructs seem unchangeable. At the same time, when we analyze the social circumstances of "natural" experiences over time, we can see how the meanings of social constructs change. This analysis challenges "facts" that we take for granted, such as the idea that women are inherently better caretakers than men.

Intersectionality

When Kimberlé Crenshaw coined the term *intersectionality* in 1989,[5] she meant its use to be as an analytical method to explain and resist oppressions shaped by multiple identities. Crenshaw was not the first scholar to discuss structural multiple and overlapping identities. She drew from and contributed to the scholarship of multicultural feminist theorists and activists. Women's studies scholars and activists emphasized the importance of avoiding one category to explain oppression and resistance. In the late 1970s and 1980s, women of color, lesbians, and working-class women revolutionized feminist theory when they theorized about the differences among women across race, class, sexuality, and national boundaries. Collections such as *This Bridge Called My Back*[6] and *Home Girls: A Black Feminist Anthology*[7] challenged mainstream definitions of sisterhood, which declared white, middle-class, heterosexual women's experiences as universal.[8] Gloria Anzaldua's *Borderlands*[9] and Chandra Mohanty's now-classic essay in which she revisits *Under Western Eyes*[10] explained the experience of mixed ethnicities and nationalities and demonstrated the importance of challenging the epistemo-logical construction of structures themselves.

Just as intersectionality has been celebrated, it has also been misused and misunderstood.[11] In 2009, at the annual meeting of the National Women's Studies Association (NWSA), Kimberlé Crenshaw and sociologist Bonnie Thornton Dill reminded conference participants that intersectionality is a theory and method grounded in emancipation. They argued that previously subordinated experiences reveal new, emancipatory knowledge. I do not use the word *emancipation* lightly. Intersectionality is freeing: it frees individuals to name systematic oppressions and privileges, it frees activists to seek solidar-ity with other groups, and it frees scholars to precisely explain social life. At the same time, intersectionality is not intersectionality if it does not attend to the dynamics of race. Crenshaw and Dill's session at NWSA clarified that intersectionality without race is a neoliberal project because it does not attend to how race historically and currently shapes social and economic life, grants privileges, and creates oppressions. Not seeing race could potentially "white-wash" social analyses—that is, act as if race does not matter. Paula Rothen-berg[12] and other scholars of whiteness remind us that race always matters; we just have to see how social and economic privilege yielded by race functions as "normal." In nursing, meanings of professional care have been ideologically whitewashed. Professional, academic, and administrative mandates create the idea that care is a universal value and nurses can and should provide the same care to all patients regardless of their social and economic backgrounds.

As a conceptual tool, intersectionality theory avoids universal and essen-tialist characterizations of gender such as theories that suggest all women are naturally caring.[13] It does not reduce explanations of oppression and privilege to a linear, additive model—for example, all black women experience more oppression at work than all white women. Linear, additive explanations pri-oritize one structure, such as gender, as the primary explanatory factor of social phenomena. In this case, because gender is analyzed first, it suggests absolutely that women experience more oppression at work than men and that minority race just makes this gendered oppression worse. Linear, addi-tive models assume that there is one true explanation of oppression and fail, for example, to recognize that men of color, gay men, immigrant men, trans men, or differently abled men might experience oppression at work. Instead, intersectionality theory considers how the specific interplay of multiple struc-tures at any one time and place can change assumed meanings of social ideas, values, and acts.

Scholars who use intersectionality theory to study sociology must stay true to how and when their categories emerge in the analysis, or we run the risk of erroneously including categories simply for the sake of inclusiveness. It is perhaps ironic but true that a scholar's attempts to be inclusive could result in statements of false universals. Scholars may conflate distinct effects or mask salient patterns in their data by attempting to analyze all possible relationships, rather than the ones that specifically emerge from the data.[14] One way to precisely analyze the influence of multiple social constructs on inequalities is to use intersectionality to inform conceptual strategies and research design.[15]

One of the most compelling arguments for the use of intersectionality is by sociologist Patricia Hill Collins. In her 1999 essay "Moving beyond Gender: Intersectionality and Scientific Knowledge," Collins suggests that we use intersectionality to challenge the process of knowledge making in sociology, just as sociologists of gender called for a study of gender within the discipline of sociology decades before. Scholars who use intersectionality are equipped to analyze how social identities construct values and ideas that we sometimes take for granted as natural and universally experienced by people. Collins's call to use intersectionality to change knowledge requires scholars to not just analyze the ideological and structural effects of the intersections of social identities but also examine how these relations inform the process of how people make meaning or understand social life. As Collins writes, "Those who have power (which means those who produce knowledge) determine which categories are deemed normal and which are deviant."[16] Although in this particular article Collins uses intersectionality to challenge feminist critiques of science, I am interested here in her grander aim: the use of intersectionality for the production of sociological and women's and gender studies knowledge. Professional intimacy changes meanings of intimate care in nursing because it changes how we understand the function, use, and negotiation of intimacy in professional care work as social and changeable depending on the identities of people involved.

Today, intersectionality is used in various disciplines including law, sociology, women's and gender studies, psychology, political science, and health sciences. Scholars who apply intersectionality to care work show that intersections of race, gender, and nationality change our understandings of care work, especially for immigrant domestic and service workers.[17] Scholars tend to label their use of intersectionality as an intersectional approach. This demonstrates how intersectionality is a means to analyze the impact of multiple identities in social interaction, ideologies, and institutions. It explains the influence of structural privilege and oppression and multiple sites of power and calls for accountability and other politics of social justice.[18] In other words, intersectionality is used as a research method, a theory to explain social life, a literary device, and a politic. I agree with Michelle Tracy Berger and Kathleen Guidroz, who argue that scholars who seek to understand social life should engage with intersectionality as a new "social literacy" and continue to debate, theorize, and apply intersectionality to the issues they study.[19]

Proponents of intersectionality agree that intersectionality can be conceptualized many ways: as a theory, a methodological approach, a context to situate people's experience, and a lens to act. It is here that I share my inspiration and my goal for the use of intersectionality in this book. After years of thinking about research and programming that captures the impact of multiple identities, I also claim intersectionality as my methodological and theoretical approach. What I mean is that I use intersectionality as a way to develop my research question, shape my design, think through power dynamics, and explain the social, economic, and symbolic meanings of everyday life. To study nursing care today, we cannot separate social constructs of race, gender, sexuality, and nationality because individuals do not live—identify, perceive, and practice—these experiences separately.

Intersections of Gender, Race, and Nationality in Nursing

Much of the nurses' intimate work I observed was behind closed doors in a patient's room. These interactions were invisible to the rest of the unit because they occurred in private when a nurse provided intimate care for a patient. How I analyze these experiences further highlights intersections of race, gender, and nationality as social constructs that inform the meaning of intimate care. These examples also illustrate how the relationship between meanings of social constructs and meanings of care affects the work of a nurse of color:

> I walked into the conference room to find Mary, an African American night nurse with twenty-eight years of experience, finishing her charting. I introduced myself, and she seemed very interested in the study. She told me she has worked in critical care, home health, and med-surg. We talked for some time. I explained the purpose of my research. She immediately shared a story about an elderly white male patient who told her that she reminded him of his mammy! She was upset by this, especially because she was taking care of his private body parts at the time. She felt demeaned but just continued caring for him. What else could she do?! She told me that nurses deal with these things by venting to each other.[20]

It is no coincidence that this patient thought "mammy" when he saw Mary. When seeing a black woman, the patient drew on a familiar image to him, what sociologist Patricia Hill Collins calls a "controlling image," at the intersection of race and gender. Controlling images are rooted in historical economic and social relations and still have power today because they justify and normalize discrimination and inequality. Collins explains:

> The first controlling image applied to U.S. Black women is that of the mammy—the faithful, obedient domestic servant. Created to justify the economic exploitation of house slaves and sustained to explain Black women's long standing restriction to domestic service, the mammy image represents the normative yardstick to evaluate all Black women's behavior. By loving, nurturing, and caring for her White children and "family" better than her own, the mammy symbolizes the dominant group's perceptions of the ideal Black female relationship to elite White male power.[21]

When Mary's patient told Mary that she reminded him of his mammy, he likely meant no harm to her. He likely sought closeness and familiarity with his caregiver in a time that was scary for him. More important to this book, however, is that in order for him to make this connection to his nurse he needed two things simultaneously: first, he needed to have the controlling image of "mammy" socially available to him, and second, he needed to want to feel close to his nurse. This need for closeness in an otherwise professional setting is the impetus for the professional intimacy that I explain in this book.

Nurses provide professional intimacy to patients because patients need them to be both professional and intimate; however, the labor (for the nurse) and the experience (for the patient) of professional intimacy is a social phenomenon that is shaped by social constructs of identity. Connecting Mary to his mammy likely made hospital care feel safer for her patient, but it also makes invisible the skill and knowledge needed to provide professionally intimate care. Moreover, it both racializes and genders Mary into a figure who is not professional, but someone who is naturally subordinate to the patient as a white man. Controlling images are controlling because they make oppressions normal and an inevitable part of life. They serve to mask real social conditions by justifying discrimination and oppression. The controlling image of "mammy" makes it seem like women of color are naturally subordinate to white men, white women, and men of color. This image is one example of how the intersection of race and gender informs the process of professionally intimate care and the work experience for women of color nurses.

Inequalities in nursing result from various combinations of controlling images about gender, race, and nationality because nursing demographics include men, women, people of color, white people, and immigrant nurses. Immigrant nurses also experience the impact of controlling images. For example, in 1999 recruiters in the United Kingdom justified the Philippines as the "natural" place to start recruiting nurses since Filipinas are "inherently" caring.[22] Racial, xenophobic, and gender inequalities persist in nursing today in part because women of color are simultaneously stereotyped as inherently less professional than white women and as naturally better caregivers. Their professional care work is more likely to be invisible when compared to that of their peers.[23]

It is important to be clear about which identities are functioning and which are not when using intersectionality to study inequalities.[24] I observed nurses and administrators conflate one identity for another when explaining inequalities in patient care. Nurse Director Anita explained how a patient's xenophobia affected his perceptions of care. Interestingly, she identified the patient's request as a race problem:

> I've had patients call me into their room and tell me—I mean, not too long ago, a man that told me he wanted an American nurse! And I paused; where is he going with this? And I happened to think of who was taking care of him. It was a nurse who I think is from Nigeria, or Africa or somewhere. Another nurse who was covering her was from Taiwan; the patient care technician who was working that day was from Eastern Europe somewhere—she has an accent. She's white, but she has an accent. And man, I suddenly realized where he was going with this, and I said, "I'm sorry sir; I can't make nursing assignments based on race." And I said I'd be in a whole lot of trouble. You know, I just wanted him to get the message—that I wasn't changing his—the assignment, and if he was truly upset about the care the nurse is giving, that would be one thing.

When Anita heard that a patient wanted an "American nurse" she began to imagine which of her nurses currently had this patient. Her first thoughts went to nationality. She said, "It was a nurse who I think is from Nigeria, or Africa or somewhere." When the patient complained, she sorted nurses in her mind based on nationality. Then she began to think of other social identifiers: accent and race. "She's white, but she has an accent." It was perhaps in this moment when Anita transferred nationality into race. She thought nationality first but then realized that the complaint had to do with race because "she suddenly realized where he was going with this." When she said she could not make assignments based on race, Anita implied that the patient was being racist. An intersectional approach would begin to explain both the patient's request and Anita's response as statements that were not just about race or about nationality but, rather, ones that occurred at the unique intersection of race and nationality.

Nurses of color described to me the ways in which racist and xenophobic attitudes of patients influenced how others perceived their labor. Mia, an experienced Filipina nurse, explained how patients focused on race when they distinguished good care from bad care. She said, "It happens! And you're not the one who did it but you are the one who gets remembered because of your color, and you are the one who gets reprimanded." Mia described how a patient complained about her bedside manner despite what Mia identifies as her "gentle" demeanor. The patient confused Mia with a white patient care technician who was "rough" and "somewhat rude." When the patient complained about unnecessary rough treatment the next day, the patient identified Mia as the offender. Mia explained:

One of the techs has this heavy [Eastern European] accent, and she is white. She is rough with the patients, and the way she communicates is not the best. Her tone of voice is kind of rude sometimes. I am always gentle. Guess who gets reported as being very rude? Do you think the white skin is going to be reported? No, it's me. And it was not me! And I thought, "Okay. What they remember is your color, and they don't care what you [actually] did. You are the one that is going to get reported." And it is not that one time. It happens a lot. [*Her voice lowered and she looked away as she said this.*]

In this case, Mia's skin color trumped the other nurses' accent (as an indicator of nationality) when the patient determined who to report as "rude." I found that perceptions and practices of nationality also constructed professional intimacy. Nurses from other countries described how white, American patients trusted them less than they did white, American nurses. I also observed white patients express their fears and anxieties about their illness through xenophobic attitudes, behaviors, and harassment that focused on nurses' languages and accents. Nurses of color also described how patients of color—especially those from Latin American countries—seemed to trust them more. Considering the impact of nationality on the process of professionally intimate care is important because nurses do not always personally or professionally benefit from international nurse migration.[25] At the same time, traditionally marginalized patients of color felt safer with immigrant nurses and other nurses of color.

Commercialized Intimacy: Intimate Care as Global Enterprise

Together, nurses and patients structure quality health care as a social interaction, which is influenced by the intersections of multiple identities. However, nursing is not just social; it is a transnational enterprise driven in large part by money. Hospitals, health-care organizations, and entire countries structure care by what Arlie Hochschild calls the "commercialization of feelings in a global exchange of care,"[26] which focuses on profit and a shortage of nurses.[27] Through transnational exchanges of nurses and other care workers, care is exported and imported, bought and sold in local hospitals, and transformed in global systems. Like other commodities, the production of care occurs in a series of phases at different locations in different parts of the world.[28]

In health care, it is the training and education of nurses that in part produces intimate care. A Marxist analysis of the production of nurses helps to illuminate how developing countries lose their investments when they educate nurses only to see them emigrate to more economically advanced nations. This surplus value of care at the first phase of production (the nurse's home country) generates profit for investors such as immigrant nurse recruitment organizations. Therefore, imported and exported on a global scale, intimate care labor forms a chain of production that contributes to capitalist wealth but receives little acknowledgment in mainstream social and economic arenas.[29] Developed nations such as the United States, the United Kingdom, and Canada recruit nurses through formalized "managed migration" agreements from developing nations or "nations in transition" such as India, Cuba, and the Philippines.[30] These global exchanges of intimate care result from the economic push and pull factors in various countries.[31] These include employment shortages in exporting countries and nursing labor shortages in importing counties.[32]

The pull factors are a shortage of care workers and care providers in Western nations. The nursing shortage in the United States is well documented. The U.S. Department of Health and Human Services (DHHS) reports that forty-four states and the District of Columbia will face serious nursing shortages by the year 2020. In 2002, U.S. president George W. Bush signed the Nurse Reinvestment Act. This legislation provided federal funds to hospitals, universities, and other health organizations to recruit, educate, and retain nurses and nursing students in the United States. In July 2004, DHHS granted $15.5 million to expand the nation's supply of qualified, minority nurses. Another proposed solution to the nursing shortage is Magnet hospitals.[33] Inspired by efforts of the American Nurses Association to create better work environments for nurses, Magnet hospitals recruit and retain nurses by reorganizing work environments and decision-making processes. They formalize decision-making processes that include all levels of staff, expect nurses to continue their education and share knowledge with other nurses, and support nurses' autonomy.[34]

Although many hospitals and associations use a combination of strategies, the primary solution to the nursing shortage in the United States has been the training, recruitment, and immigration of foreign-born nurses. Sociologist Catherine Choy shows how the United States established hospital training programs in the Philippines in the early 1900s as a way to establish low-cost labor and acculturate the Filipino population to American standards.[35] Several recent nursing relief acts (from 1989 through 1999) provided immigrant nurses special status and consideration, extending their visas to accommodate health-care crises in the United States. These acts stemmed from the Immigration and Nationality Act of 1965, which liberalized immigration from formerly restricted areas such as Korea and the Philippines. Filipinas took advantage of the U.S. Exchange Visitor Program. The United States developed this program to improve post–Cold War relations, but it also provided the country with low-cost labor. Immigrants received work stipends for two years, after which they would return to their home countries. The government waived this residency requirement for "certain" nurses in 1970, which prompted the Philippines government to actively promote nurse employment contracts with the United States. Because the act opened up opportunities for immigration from formerly restricted countries, it became more likely that governments—especially those in debt—would respond and become more dependent on human and other product-export-oriented economies rather than focus on their own internal development.

In 2003, The International Council of Nurses (ICN), a federation of 125 national nursing associations representing millions of nurses worldwide, initiated the Global Nursing Workforce Project to examine the global nursing shortage and nursing migration patterns. In March 2004, the Project produced its first report, "The Global Shortage of Registered Nurses: An Overview of Issues and Actions."[36] This report named international migration as one of three critical challenges faced by policy makers, personnel, and advocates who work to provide access to safe, adequate, and affordable health care in all regions around the world. The report also advocates for an increase in wages among other solutions to help with nurse retention and recruitment. Hospitals also benefit from the exchange of care because invisible and unrecognized, intimate care is an inexpensive commodity that results in satisfied patients and families. National governments benefit from the economic exchange of care; Western nations lure nurses from poorer countries, and developing nations receive financial assistance for training and education efforts.

Managed health care and hospital restructuring in the United States provide another point of entry for discussing the commodification of intimacy in nursing care.[37] Nurses know that illness and injury are always scary, but in a time of managed care, thoughts of illness and injury are frightening at best and economically impossible at worst. Nurses want to do their best for their patients, but just do not have the time.[38] Many nurses work more than three or four twelve-hour shifts per week because they need the money and administrators need to fill vacancies stemming from the still-persistent nursing shortage. The nursing shortage has had profound effects on hospital nursing at the levels of practice and administration. To the current nurse, the nursing shortage means exhausting and seemingly never-ending shifts. To the nurse administrator, the nursing shortage means agonizing over unfilled nurses' jobs, losing nurses to other institutions, and overburdening current nurses with too many hours and too many patients. To the future nurse, however, the nursing shortage means job opportunities and security. As a result, many more people are entering the nursing profession for financial reasons and not out of some sense of a "calling" to the profession. This does not, of course, mean there are not still those nurses who enter the field out of a love for the job.

Unfortunately, for all nurses, managed health care means too much paperwork, too many patients, and too little time. I watched nurses chart all day but still not have time to document the intimate care they provided. These nurses were often frustrated in their desire to intimately connect with their patients and by the restrictions placed on their time by what they felt was bureaucratic paper pushing. Nurses cared all the time, but this work went unnoticed—in part because they did not have the time to document it but also because other medical staff saw them as unofficial managers of information, not as care providers. For example, even though nurses carefully documented every change in each patient's condition in a chart, doctors and other medical staff often did not take the time to look through the chart. Instead, they turned to nurses for quick information on a patient's current status. Nurses told me that other medical personnel learned to expect this information from nurses, information that will help them do their jobs more quickly and efficiently. These expectations helped to solidify an additional work requirement for the nurse. The nurse was responsible not only for caring for patients and documenting this care but also for being available to transmit to other medical personnel and to family members information about any patient at a moment's notice. In essence, the nurse was both providing and coordinating patient care.[39] What was further burdensome was that the nurse rarely had the authority to talk about care and deferred to the physician on call.

Most of the administrators directly experienced the nursing shortage as an economic issue in nursing because although they worked in a Magnet hospital they often pulled on temporary reserves to fill the ranks. Although this was a midsize hospital with approximately 250 beds, there was a staffing and resource department wholly devoted to making sure that units were staffed. In addition, nurse directors were familiar with the burdens of managed care policies and understood how these policies negatively affected bedside care. When it came to the relationship between intimate labor and the provision of quality health care, however, administrators were unaware, almost naive. For example, when she decided to check in with patients in their rooms, an administrator realized that working with patients "means you just all of a sudden, you feel like you are a part of their family. You feel so drawn to what is happening to them and emotionally involved." When she saw patients, it was mostly because they "emotionally just need to vent and afterwards, after you listen, they don't want other actions." When I asked the hospital president if he thought nursing was intimate, he responded by saying that patients feel vulnerable and that this vulnerability requires an intimate connection. Experienced nurses knew that taking the time to sit with patients on their beds, for example, translated to patients that their nurses care about them more personally than if the nurse "stood at the edge of the bed, kind of poised to be on the way out."[40] Nurses work hard to be intimately caring; they use emotions to give care that seems authentic and also maintain professional boundaries at the same time.[41]

Two important sociological concepts help reveal the explicit connection among emotions, bodies, and the economy in professional intimacy. These are Arlie Russell Hochschild's concept of emotional labor and Miliann Kang's concept of body labor.[42] As concepts (also introduced in the beginning of this book), emotional labor and body labor explain how commercialized intimacy becomes labor for the worker, constitutes part of the purchase for the client, and increases profit for the employer. In addition to and essentially as part of quality health care, patients receive positive emotional and physical interactions from nurses. This labor is invisible, not counted, and not paid for. However, because it is designed to invoke positive feelings in patients, patients may feel entitled to behaving in ways that, while comfortable for them, are discomforting for the nurse. The hospital makes money because it can offer patients a positive experience without having to compensate their nurses for the labor of producing and sustaining positive emotions.

I observed Angie, an African nurse, prepare medication for her white male patient in his room. As she smoothly inserted the carefully mixed concoction into his arm, he remarked to her, "That's slick. I wish you could show all of them how to do that." Angie responded, "Yes, it makes a difference if you mix it before." He then asked, "Were you kidding before when you said you had to find a vein?" She kept up with what she was doing but murmured, "No." The patient had a concerned expression on his face and seemed nervous. He said, "You sounded angry." She did not overly reassure him but faintly shook her head "no." In addition to concentrating on the IV, Angie helped produce a feeling of security in her patient by verbally engaging him while she completed a medical procedure that requires close attention. Perhaps more important, Angie deftly negotiated her patient's need to feel secure in her expertise as well as his need for her to not be "angry." This interaction occurred because Angie knew how to simultaneously provide medical care and evoke a feeling of trust in her patient. An experienced nurse, Angie knew that providing quality health care meant that she simultaneously reassure her patient and successfully administer the IV medication.

Professional intimacy differs from emotional labor in part because nurses choose this labor to comfort their patients, build trust with them, and make the execution of their other tasks run more smoothly. Hospitals do not coerce them to do it. In addition, unlike emotional labor, professional intimacy explains how nurses create and sustain intimate care through the work of their bodies and how this work is influenced by social constructs of race, gender, sexuality, and nationality. To help analyze these patterns of body labor, I draw on Miliann Kang's study of three Korean nail salons in New York City.[43] In her study, Kang conceptualizes body labor as work that includes both physical and emotional management and changes between women from different race and class backgrounds and according to the socioeconomic conditions of the neighborhoods in which they work. Interactions between the manicurist and the client capitalize on gender, racial, and ethnic stereotypes of Korean immigrants (for example, the stereotype that Korean women are naturally docile and more adept at paying attention to detail) and enforces the privilege of white customers (for example, the notion that rich, white women are entitled to pampering and emotional attention).

Consider the ways that Angie, the nurse I introduced previously, bodily and emotionally managed her patient during my observations of her labor:

I followed Angie into a semiprivate room. At the southernmost side of the room is a very frail, thin, elderly white man in bed. Sitting in chairs around him are his wife and daughter. He needs to walk but is not responding to Angie's voice from the end of the bed. Angie maneuvered herself closer to the patient's face, bent down, and looked into his eyes. She repeated his name and her request to walk him. He ignored her. His daughter dryly smiled at his resistance. It is as if she knows her father well and knows that he hears Angie but is choosing to not respond. Angie continued to repeat his name, gentle but firm. The patient finally responded and said, "I don't care." Angie responded, "I care!" She walked to the other side of the bed and carefully moved his legs down.[44]

In this case, Angie manipulated her body position to intimately connect with her patient, persisted verbally, and then reinforced the intimacy of the interaction by exclaiming, "I care!" Angie drew on her long experience of negotiating her patients' physical postures, emotional presentations, and intense feelings to help them receive the medical care she knew they needed. As an experienced nurse, Angie knew that this labor will help facilitate quality health care. She understands that the caring interaction often begins with a patient's fear and resistance and that she had to work through this fear to do her job. In the rest of this book, I analyze how securing intimate trust, negotiating intimate conflict, and participating in collective intimate strategies draw on emotional and body labor at intersections of gender, race, and nationality. This analysis contributes both to social meanings of intimate care and to how this intimacy is an economic exchange.

The nurse directors I observed and interviewed offered contradictory views of the intimate care-versus-money dilemma. Although all directors agreed care work was specialized labor, each also described care as a natural trait or a moral act when they speculated whether or not a nurse was a good nurse. Without my prompting, nurse directors consistently explained how they assessed bedside nurses by their reasons for entering the profession. Nurse directors expressed fear that new nurses were in it only for the money and did not feel a moral call to nurse. Nurse Director Peggy described her concern about nurses who saw nursing as only a job. She valued the nurses who talked about not needing their salaries:

I expect my nurses to show a passion. It is disheartening to me over the holidays just to see the nurses competing for the higher dollar because they weren't doing it for the right reason, but it was a revitalizing moment when one of my nurses said she'd be willing to work extra hours. She said, "Peggy, I don't do it for the money. I don't do nursing for the money. Do you need help or not?" She goes, "I'm not worried about the bonus; I'm not worried about that." She stepped up, and it was from her heart.

Peggy was not alone. Many of the nurse administrators I talked with yearned for a fantastical time when nurses felt called to nursing and did not focus on money or work conditions. This fantastical image of the good nurse fails to reflect a substantial history of professionalization and also limits nursing to a sacred calling rather than professional work that requires knowledge and expertise. Moreover, this idea that "good nurses do not decide to become nurses because it pays well" is further complicated by the international economic conditions of health care, which include the power of health management organizations, the problem of nursing shortages, and the solution of nurse emigration and immigration.

Directors described nurses who do not need money as good nurses, implying that those who do are bad nurses. When asked why individuals choose nursing as a career over other jobs, Molly, a nurse director responded, "Most nurses do it for a couple of reasons now: it is good money or it is a true calling and they do not care about the finances." Frowning, showing concern about the state of nursing, Anita admitted that "there is fierce competition between hospitals" and that "most of the reasons people do not accept jobs are over pay." Anita also worries that "vice presidents and nurse directors sometime along the way have forgotten what it means to really care. We've been in meetings, and they talk about customer service, and I think they forget what it takes to be a nurse." How these directors force a discrepancy between wages and a desire to care for patients is a binary "setup" similar to the ones that Patricia Hill Collins describes in her analysis of controlling images of African American women: "In such thinking difference is defined in oppositional terms. One part is not simply different from its counterpart; it is inherently opposed to its 'other.' Whites and Blacks, males and females, thought and feeling are not complementary counterparts—they are fundamentally different entities related only through their definition as opposites."[45]

Framed in opposition, it seems that intimacy cancels out money and money tarnishes intimacy. This thinking contributes to the invisibility of care work because it prevents an explanation of how care is produced through research, teaching, and clinical work. How nurse directors frame care in opposition to money also suggests that at any given time one or the other is most important and has more value in the experience of health care: "Finally because oppositional binaries rarely represent different but equal relation-ships, they are inherently unstable. Tension may be temporarily relieved by subordinating one half of the binary to the other. Thus Whites rule Blacks, men dominate women, reason is thought superior to emotion in ascertain-ing truth, facts supersede opinion in evaluating knowledge, and subjects rule objects."[46]

Through her discussion of binaries, Collins reveals how a definition of quality health care in terms of money or care is ultimately reductive. Position-ing money and care in opposition suggests that nurses and administrators disagree about what is best for patients. This was absolutely not the case in the hospital I studied; each nurse and administrator I spoke with consistently considered the needs of patients. Most of the administrators in the hospi-tal were also nurses and had at one point in their careers worked bedside. Although some directors feared that other directors lost sight of care in the interest of money, all of the directors I interviewed emphasized how much they valued care. When administrators value care as an ideal, they do not necessarily recognize or measure the labor of care: "I think that it's probably, um, one of the biggest aspects of giving care to a patient who has entrusted care to you at a very vulnerable time in their lives. The degree of, um, giving of oneself and being, um, open with a patient is hard to articulate. I'm stum-bling on what that would mean. The emotional aspect, I think, is such a high ratio of what happens at the bedside."[47]

Intrigued by how nurse directors assessed the quality of bedside nurses, I began to ask how the hospital formally assesses the quality of care it provides. When I asked one nursing administrator how the hospital measures care, she laughed ironically and told me, "We do not." When I asked how the hospital staff knows that care is accomplished, she and other administrators started talking about patient satisfaction forms. As they were discharged, each patient was asked to complete an evaluation of their stay. Nurse directors and other hospital administrators used these forms to demonstrate to the community and other investors that the hospital values care. My analysis of patient satisfaction reports revealed that patients primarily described care by emphasizing two things: the kindness of their nurses and the quality of food. Nurse directors ironically laughed when I asked them about assessing care, because they already knew what I had discovered when I studied the patient satisfaction forms: the actual care work of nurses was not assessed and was not recognized.

Although administrators—even former bedside nurses—appreciated nurses who were caring, they could not articulate the process of care or how nurses strategically negotiated intimacy with their patients to ensure quality health care. Although the patient satisfaction form asks only one question about nurses, the hospital president insisted to me that patient satisfaction (forms and other communications) measured care:

> It measures caring. It doesn't measure clinical care. We have measures of clinical care. It measures caring by showing how people are communicating with each other. When they are responsible, when they address them by name, when they explain to them what is going on. People feel cared for. People complain the most about a lack of response to call lights. The caring is being explained to—translating for the doctors; that's the nurture. There's no expression for it in hospital work. Patients care about three things: cleanliness, kindness, and good food. The kindness is really that element of human compassion and communication and things like that.

I would argue, however, that patient satisfaction does not measure care so much as it measures customer service. As the hospital president said to me, "You are getting people at the worst moment. We place a lot of emphasis on customer satisfaction. It is something we track and something we report. We place a lot of emphasis on that we want people to have a highly satisfied stay here." Although directors used these forms to assess how well nurses cared for patients, patients most often discussed food and noise and used words like "service" in the patient satisfaction forms I read and in the comments I heard. This use is one way that patients and administrators conflated patient satisfaction with care of patients.

Although it was not explicitly stated by administrators to them, bedside nurses knew it was their responsibility to keep patients satisfied as customers. As Celia, a new nurse, described, "We act like a five-star hotel. Our patients are now customers. They're here for care. In my eyes, it's a privilege. They can treat you like shit, and you're supposed to just take it. It takes some of your validity away as a caregiver. I think when they get home, what they're going to remember is that they didn't get their way, complaining whether or not they get chocolate or strawberry [ice cream]."

The patients' and administrators' focus on satisfaction not only demeaned the validity of care work; it also failed to accurately measure skill and expertise. Nurses faced a conundrum when required to keep patients "satisfied" during their hospital stay: the quality of their labor was measured by the happiness of their patients, yet a nurses' job required him or her to perform acts that necessarily dissatisfy the patient—withholding food, repeatedly drawing blood, prioritizing other patients, and the like. While nurses and administrators prioritized the patient's perspective during care, patients could not always know what was best for them or know the obligations that nurses had to other patients. The expectations that patients and family members have of nurses also conflicted with those of hospital administrators who track nursing work through charting and other standardized documentation that record medications, orders, procedures, and vital signs.[48]

The patient satisfaction forms I reviewed did not measure intimacy, trust, or the conflict that could result from increased familiarity with bedside nurses. In addition, a feeling of trust did not occur naturally between nurses and patients and between nurses and patients' families. Although intimate care is a significant commodity in the global marketplace, social scientists, feminist scholars, and individual care workers know that care work is invisible; it is misunderstood, taken for granted, and undervalued, and when it is paid at all, it is underpaid. The separation of intimacy from profit and wages is false because quality health care requires both elements. Moreover, the invisibility of the relationship between intimate care and money maintains the myth that being caring is a natural personality trait and not labor.

Patients and their families brought fear of illness and injury, fear of the medical system, and fear of others to the hospital with them. Although many nurses were hesitant to use the word *intimacy* to describe their work, I observed them strategically using intimacy to negotiate their patients' discomforts and fears throughout their stay in the hospital. Experienced nurses in my study created, perceived, developed, and experienced intimate care in nursing to build and maintain a trusting relationship with patients.

The three chapters that follow describe and analyze the labor of professional intimacy. Taken individually, these chapters exemplify how nurses professionally negotiated intimate labor and how these labors changed in various social and economic contexts. These chapters should also be read as interrelated, because each describes a stage of professional intimacy that informs the next. In the first stage of intimate trust, I show how nurses worked to gain the trust of patients. This labor was invisible to patients and family members often on purpose to help patients feel safe in a fear-provoking environment. As some patients felt an increasing sense of comfort and familiarity with their nurses, they also developed a sense of entitlement to them. These entitlements resulted in various emotional and bodily intimate conflicts that nurses negotiated as part of their nursing labor. Whether or not these conflicts were sexualized (some were and some were not), they were all intimate and resulted from commodifications of intimacy in the context of commercialized intimacy. Nurses responded to intimate conflict in various ways by redeveloping trust with their patients. They returned to intimate trust strategies even if it meant exploitative labor conditions for them. They did this because they keenly believed that trust was critical to their patients' well-being and ability to receive quality health care.

3

Catheters, Communications, and Intimate Trust

Getting a catheterization is one of the many ordinary hospital procedures that is intimate for the patient but not for the nurse. Instead, the intimacy in acts of care—such as carefully inserting a catheter—is mundane intimate labor. I have used the act of giving and receiving a catheter to help illustrate why nurses need their patients to trust them. On a continual basis, when patients trust their nurses, it is easier for them to receive quality health care. New nurses are not prepared to handle intimacy, but experienced nurses know that the way patients trust them is through intimacy. Over time, nurses develop strategies to build intimacy with patients to facilitate trust. I analyze these strategies as invisible work that is influenced by social meanings of multiple identities.

The quality care of patients requires that patients trust their nurses. As I said previously, I name the work that senior nurses are *already* doing as professional intimacy and argue that professional intimacy is what fosters and maintains this trust. Unlike personal intimacies, trust between patients and nurses rarely feels natural to the nurse even if it does for the patient. Patients and family members are often scared when they first enter the hospital. Patients feel vulnerability, physical pain, and mixed emotions—fear, anxiety, depression, and hope. They wear hospital gowns that sometimes do not cover their entire bodies, have strangers walking in and out of their rooms at all hours of the day, and usually have little technical knowledge of what is happening to them. At times, they have no control over their bodies or emotions. Experienced bedside nurses know that patients feel emotionally and physically exposed in the hospital. They provide quality care in part by facilitating a culture of intimacy, which helps patients feel safe and comfortable.

I listened to nurses describe how patients were fearful when they entered the hospital and did not trust the health-care process. Because trust did not occur naturally among nurses and patients and their families, nurses created a sense of familiarity to increase trust and ease patients' fears. This is the work of intimate trust. From my interviews, I discovered that although nurses knew that intimacy benefited patients and their family members, nurse administrators expressed discomfort when discussing the role of intimacy in their professional work.[1] Some nurses, especially those new to the profession, expressed shock at the degree of intimacy required and discomfort when they learned intimacy was part of the job. Other nurses were clear that they did not consider nursing personally intimate but said that patients perceived their care as intimate. Still others defined intimacy as necessary to patient healing. Regardless of how nurses identified or felt about intimacy as an idea, all nurses discussed how they used intimacy in their professional practice. Individually and collectively, nurses built a culture of intimacy to increase the comfort of patients during their stay. In the last part of the chapter, I analyze how nurses negotiated trust and familiarity with patients and families across boundaries and perceptions of gender, race, and nationality. How intimate trust changes at these intersections changes the meaning of care and can contribute to inequalities in nursing.

The Importance of Intimacy in Professional Care Work

To many bedside nurses, intimate connections contributed to healing, especially when they thought of intimacy the way they imagined their patients did. While nurses thought intimacy was important for care, nurses did not necessarily experience giving care as an intimate experience *for them*. Amy, an experienced nurse, told me, "Nursing is fast paced. You are not spending a long time with each patient—well, not on days [day shift] where we're usually running around in and out of five rooms." As a hospital nurse, Amy did not feel that she had the time to develop close, intimate relationships with her patients. Jason, another experienced nurse, agreed that time was important to developing intimacy. He acknowledged that although patients and nurses were emotionally accessible to each other, he did not consider this availability to be intimate:

I think [patients] let you in, and you let them in for hours or days. And that's the difference. If it is intimacy, it's so brief that I don't even feel like I miss them when they're discharged home. And, to me, intimacy is almost forming a bond where you could potentially miss that person in the future.

Jason did not feel the "bond" with his patients that one might develop in a personal relationship. Nonetheless, as he continued to talk with me, Jason decided there were relationships among intimacy, time, and quality care. He explained how patients became more open with nurses as they demonstrated their skills during the patient's hospital stay. He said, "I think that a patient seeing your competencies becomes comfortable with you, and then you can become intimate with them. As they open up and you open up, you start letting down these professional obstructions."

Although Jason did not define care work as intimate, he built intimacy into his professional work because he wanted patients to heal. Jason described how intimacy in nursing was necessary for patients to feel better:

You know, even though you're looking at people's bodies, I see it as a job. I see it as work. Even though I'm getting intimate with them because they're in a gown or their pajamas, I've never even thought of it as that, oddly enough. It's the professional distance that is the difference. I'm doing this to help you and not because I want to arouse you or make you want me. I'm doing it so that you get better.

Jason made clear that intimacy in nursing was professional because its goal was to move patients toward healing. To him, maintaining professional distance helped him manage perceptions and experiences of intimacy with the patient. Bill also emphasized the need for professionalism during intimate work: "They're looking at you as, like, a professional—that you're not leaving the room talking about their body that you just viewed and the things that you just did. You're not degrading them when you leave the room." Balancing distance with closeness did not come naturally; it required skill that was developed over time. Both Jason and Bill identified that building trust requires a combination of familiarity and professionalism.

Other nurses who did not think their labor was intimate agreed that patients and family members might experience nursing care this way. Jill, a new nurse, told me, "Intimate is a strange word because there are so many different meanings, but I guess it would be a good way to describe patient care. Yes, I do think it [nursing] is intimate because you are dealing with people's bodies, and that's the most—that's personal space. We're dealing with health information, which can be embarrassing. So yes, it's very intimate. It's very special, sacred stuff." Jill said the word "intimate" could mean different things in different contexts. Initially, she hesitated when I asked her if she thought nursing work was intimate, likely because she defined intimacy in terms of personal relationships and sexuality, rather than work. She quickly reconsidered when she framed the idea of intimacy in what she imagined to be her patient's experience of nursing care. Jill resolved this tension between personal and workplace intimacy by drawing on a familiar trope: the sacredness of nursing work. As discussed in Chapter 2, there is nothing wrong with considering nursing work sacred except that it contributes to fantasies of care work that do not include labor, conflict, strategy, or skill.

Like Jason and Jill, many other nurses told me that they never thought their work was intimate until they thought about it from their patients' points of view. When I asked Lori, a new nurse, if care was intimate, she explained that it was not intimate to her, but it could be for the patient. She said, "It's not intimate, but you have to respect the patient, and you have to respect their privacy. And that's the intimate part of our job, but at the same time I don't think it's intimate. And if the patient has been in the hospital before, they know about it [lack of privacy]. If not, you know, they're a little more private. In that way it is intimate." Individuals respect the privacy of others in their homes and in their neighborhoods. In public we might step away from what we perceive to be a private conversation between two individuals, and when we do so, we assume that the individuals know each other well. The act of respecting privacy is usually reserved for the private realm. In public work, however, respect for privacy is an act of labor that considers intimate interactions from the patient's perspective. It helps to distinguish professional intimacy from other intimacies and also from other professional labors.

I remember the moment when I realized that it did not matter whether or not nurses wanted to incorporate intimacy into their work with patients. I discovered that patients sought intimacy with their nurses on a regular basis. Patients and family members contributed to the establishment of professional intimacy by seeking an intimate environment to feel safe. They drew on their own understandings of nursing to ease their tensions and fears. They disclosed personal information about themselves to nurses as a way to ensure a connection. They talked about their families, their past loves, their troubles at home, and how they became ill. They discussed their hobbies and favorite television shows. They shared their views on spirituality and their fears about death. Patients and family members talked to me, too. One patient's wife took me aside while the nurse assessed her husband and began to talk to me about how she and her husband met and fell in love. I knew she shared their love story with me as a way to connect to me, which would help her cope with her fears about her husband's illness.

Experienced nurses identified that working on people's bodies and with people's fears, comforts, pains, and hopes created intimate circumstances in their labor. Mia, an experienced Filipina nurse, described how patients reacted to her during a typical workday. "Well, they get close to you. You care for them. You want them to get better. You bond with them. They know you." In contrast to body labor and emotional labor, which are defined by profit and exploitation, Mia explained that patients felt close to her as a result of the intimate care she provided to them.

When I asked Anna, a new Latina nurse I introduced in the beginning of this book, if nursing was intimate, she responded, "Yes, because you are touching bodies, and I know this is private. This is why I reassure them, because caring for them is intimate. I want to make them comfortable." Jason also explained this connection: "And I think your intimacy grows as they trust you. And trust is a huge word, you know. There are some patients who learn that they trust these three nurses to do this particular painful procedure. Someone else comes in; they could be even better—have greater technical skill—but it doesn't matter. They don't have a rapport." Nurses who balanced this combination of familiarity and professionalism successfully practiced negotiating patients' feelings of closeness, trust, intense emotions, and bodily interactions.

When I asked Tonia, an African American nurse, if nursing was intimate, she said, "Most of it is intimate. I mean, you're touching other people's body parts. It's intimate. You've got to touch the person. You know, how uncomfortable is it for a stranger to touch you?" Carey, a new African American nurse, agreed, "And you have to be able to show compassion and love to a total stranger that, you know, you don't know. You don't know these people." Tonia and Carey framed their discussions of intimacy as a form of empathizing with patients. They saw intimacy in nursing as being not entirely personal but incorporating personal aspects. Carey described her thoughts regarding intimacy and patient care:

You are here in a bed. I'm here. You have to touch them. It's what to do. It's part of the healing. And you don't want to touch people like, "Ooh icky. I can't touch you." If they feel that way, how are they going to get better, heal? The bottom line is you have to touch them; you have to put your hands on them. It can be intimate; I think it should be. I don't think it should be so strict and rigid.

Interestingly, Anna, Carey, and Tonia are new to nursing and did not hesitate to identify the importance of intimacy in nursing, even though they felt discomfort about it. They resolved their discomfort with intimacy by evoking their patient's perspectives. This knowledge about the meaning of intimacy in nursing is in stark contrast to how nurse directors—many of whom were experienced nurses—insisted that nursing was not intimate. The nurses, however, are closest to the situation. Informed by feminist standpoint theory, I prioritize Anna's, Carey's, and Tonia's knowledge over the explanations offered by the nurse directors.

The Work of Intimacy in Professional Care Work

Most of the nurses who identified intimacy in care from the patients' perspectives were experienced nurses. In contrast, some new nurses were astonished at the level of intimacy that was part of their work. Most did not feel academically or personally prepared to handle the depth of emotion that resulted from intimate circumstances at work. As a consequence, some new nurses avoided intimacy when working with patients. Joyce described her fears and discomfort when she was too close to patients. She explained, "Like, if I'm really tired or something, while I'm talking to a patient, I'll lean against the wall. I don't sit on patient's beds. That to me is just something I'm not willing to do. And I've seen nurses do that. That's too close to me. That's too intimate. I don't like patients touching me, as terrible as that sounds. [*Laughs.*]" Joyce's laugh sounded ironic. These feelings were true for her, but they contradict the fantasy of caring described earlier in this book. When I asked Joyce why she thought not wanting patients to touch her was terrible, she explained that other nurses viewed her as a "bad" nurse, as uncaring. Joyce's story illustrates a dilemma in nursing. As a part of their labor, nurses must balance their discomforts and fears against patients' needs and, in some cases, demands.

I found that nurses could better balance patients' intimate fears and discomforts with their medical needs after they accumulated professional experience. Interestingly, many experienced nurses talked about negotiating intimacy not necessarily as a skill but as "getting back to basics" with care after they learned and practiced their medical and technical skills. At the same time experienced nurses avoided the word *skill* when talking about intimacy, they acknowledged that one could "get back to basics" only after one had accrued professional capabilities. Elizabeth, an experienced nurse, described her routine as one that new nurses did not know right away and "came with experience." Helen, also an experienced nurse, grew accustomed to working with bodies over time. She said, "That part of it, that doesn't seem intimate to me anymore. I remember when I first did it. Yeah, it was like, whoa, this is uncomfortable. Now it's not an issue. Now it becomes more intimate when you're dealing with the feelings and emotions of it." Another experienced nurse, Jody, told me that over time nurses learn how to connect with and set boundaries with patients. She said: "You just have to learn how to talk to them. It just comes with time. You know. They like to talk about their family. They like you to talk about your family. And I don't mind doing it up to a point. But I don't think they need to know where you live." What Jody meant by patients not knowing "where you live" was how she (and other experienced nurses) knew that patients would likely emotionally and physically connect with their nurses as a mundane, everyday condition of nursing care. It was her job to establish boundaries, to learn how to listen to patients, and to learn how to talk to them. Unlike new nurses, experienced nurses did not question whether patients would connect to them; they knew they would. To Jody, professional intimacy meant protecting her own boundaries while balancing her patients' medical needs with their desires.

Keeping the patients' perspectives in mind first and foremost may seem an obvious act in professional care work, but it was often what seemed most obvious that was most invisible. The things nurses did regularly were often the very things that they could not articulate.[2] Unlike other professional labors in nursing, professional intimacy is effective when it is understated. It is sometimes *not* talking, not acknowledging familiarity. Mary agreed that nursing care was intimate in the ways that it was subtle. She said:

> You are sharing something with the patients that nobody else gets to see. You're caring for them when they are in excruciating pain. I think that is most intimate because people do not want others to see them at their lowest point. And it's so funny—that's why even when you care for people, if you see them out, often you will not really talk. Because you see them at a time that no one wants to acknowledge that you saw. I took care of an employee here. He appreciated the care, talked, wrote a nice note. But afterwards he would not acknowledge me at all. And I would think, "Does he just not see me?" But it is because I took care of him at his lowest point.

In the hospital, nurses sometimes maintained professional intimacy by keeping painful and other intense interactions muted to preserve the dignity of patients and family members. Nurses told me that this increased patients' trust, but at the cost of minimizing their own labor. This aspect of professional intimacy was difficult to resolve: patients sometimes needed nurses to deny their efforts to feel trust and comfort, but when nurses met this need they exacerbated the invisibility of professional care labor. Moreover, the needs and desires of individual patients changed during their hospital stays. Nurses constantly reframed intimate conditions to best care for their patients, even when it deemphasized their labor.

Many nurses—both new and experienced—discussed the importance of taking time, first thing in the morning, to "set the day right." To "set the day right" meant that a nurse would approach each patient cheerfully, say good morning, introduce herself or himself, and ask how the patient was doing. Trixie, a new nurse, told me, "That's why when I go and see them in the morning, like, I have a conversation with them and see, and try and build, even if it's little, you know, something. So that, you know, instead of just going in there and just like, 'Okay, here's your meds. Okay, bye.' [*Laughs.*]" Elizabeth, an experienced nurse, explained, "I start when you go in and introduce yourself. Right from the get-go, I try to ask them basic need things. 'What can I do to make you feel more comfortable at the moment? Do you need a drink of water? Do you need a blanket? Would you like a washcloth to wash your face?' It is the simplest little things." This "something" that Trixie referred to is a feeling of intimate connection that would help her patients feel comfortable with her. What Elizabeth calls the "simple things" helps nurses ease into what they know is a private moment for the patient. The "simple things" bridge private intimacy to public intimacy, personal intimacy to professional intimacy. These "simple things" also help patients develop confidence in their nurses and in hospital care, more generally.

Mary, another experienced nurse, considered families when she provided "basic care": "Nobody wants to see their loved one soiled. That says to them that you don't care [about] the little, basic, daily needs. It's the little things they notice, not the big things—that they are getting all their medications. How are they situated in bed? Are they clean? Is their mouth clean? It's all those little things that tell the families that you care."

During their intimate exchanges with patients, nurses simultaneously took note of physical and medical matters such as breathing, facial expressions (to assess pain), skin coloring, and warmth of skin. The patients saw expressions of concern only while the nurses conducted medical assessments. Nurses who "set the day right" developed trust with their patients, who then became more confident in their care. These acts helped ensure that overall care progressed without difficulty. Yet, like the act of withholding familiarity with patients, facilitating intimate connections with them had to remain unacknowledged or at least unnamed for it to work. This invisibility is similar to other commercialized intimacies that capitalize on the act of making the intimate work seem natural.

Even new nurses knew how important it was for patients to have confidence in them, even if these nurses could not articulate the relationships among confidence, intimacy, trust, and quality health care as Jason did (see earlier in this chapter). Even if they felt insecure, nurses knew they needed to act with confidence so patients felt safe. Carey considered the importance of patients having confidence in her. She told me that it was her job to be sure that patients "know they're safe and that people care about them and won't hurt them." Speaking as if she were a patient, she added, "If they care about me, then I think I can trust them. I don't think they would lie to me or mislead me." When they perceived nurses to be competent, patients felt secure and were open to trusting their nurses. Many nurses discussed the importance of a neat appearance and skillful presentation to demonstrate competence to their patients. Brett asserted, "Anything that looks like you're incompetent will destroy the intimacy between you and your patient." Nurses thus needed to present a competent self to develop rapport, trust, and ultimately professional intimacy.

Nurses expressed professionalism and sympathy for the fears and vulnerabilities that prompted patients to need to feel close to them. In order for patients to believe that this sympathy was genuine, however, nurses blended a combination of emotional and body labors. Carey described how she reassured a patient who felt fearful about his heart surgery the next morning. In addition to explaining the procedures and processes that he could expect, Carey said, she also "stayed with him and massaged the back of his hand." She told me, "You can't really say he's going to be fine because you don't really know that. So I just stay there and let them [patients in general] talk about all their fears and get it all out." Carey facilitated an experience of genuine sympathy for her patient by including intimacy in her approach. She not only informed him about his upcoming procedures but also physically and emotionally reassured him.

Professional intimacy requires that nurses give attention to patients beyond medical and physical care. It also requires that they spend significant time with patients because this is what patients need and want. Nurses know that spending time with patients is important, but there is no standard guideline on how much time is necessary to accomplish trust. Instead, nurses work to understand their patients' unique personalities and then strategize on how best to negotiate these personalities.

One pattern I observed is how patients paid considerable attention to the frequency with which nurses entered and left their rooms because they (the patients) were focused on their illnesses and on getting better. Patients usually knew when their medications were due and often watched the clock closely, keeping track of the time. Nurses, on the other hand, were spread thin. They had many patients and many demands. I often noticed when nurses took a break because they rarely did so. When nurses were in patients' rooms, they were paying attention to many things at once: the patient's physical demeanor, the patient's emotional demeanor, the family's needs, IV bags and other equipment, the position of the bed, and even the cleanliness of the room. On the other hand, patients were focused only on their nurses. They watched a nurse's every move. They noticed changes in their nurses' facial expressions, tone of voice, and speed at which they moved. Mary described an interaction with a patient, "She—the patient—noticed I was focused; I was truly focused on doing something else in another room. And I came into the room, and I had to do a task, maybe hang a patient IV, and [the patient] said, 'What is wrong? Are you mad at me?' It was because I was focused on something else. It was my facial expression." Like Mary and Angie in Chapter 2, nurses who were professionally intimate with their patients knew that patients often scrutinized their nurses' words, touches, vocal tone, and body expressions and could take any of these things personally. In response, nurses worked hard to account for their behaviors, their personal expressions, and changes in their routines as well as those of other staff members.

One aspect of nurses' work that changed often was their routine. Nurses told me that some nurse educators encouraged them to avoid sharing their routines with patients because it could potentially add extra work for the nurse. Educators warned that if nurses were honest with their patients, they might inadvertently encourage patients to monitor them (and the clock) more closely, which could make patients appear more demanding to them. Carey told me she learned to avoid telling patients when she planned to go back to their rooms, although patients consistently asked her when she would return to them. "And that was something we learned in nursing school. Don't give them a timeline. Don't say, 'I'll be back in five minutes.' Guaranteed they are looking at their watch, and at five minutes they'll be on the call light." According to these educators, it may be better to be vague with patients because specificity could establish a dynamic that would cause patients to experience undue stress. Nurses could help patients avoid this stress if they did not set up time expectations that could likely be unmet because of circumstances beyond their control.

Although nurses might save time, potential conflict, and undue stress on the part of patients by withholding their routines from patients, experienced nurses disagreed with this advice. They maintained a routine to keep their work organized and efficient but constantly shifted this routine to prioritize the needs of some patients over others, depending on each patient's situation. They felt that by sharing changes in their routines with their patients, they established a mutual accountability that fostered closeness and trust. When I asked Mary, an experienced nurse, if she informed patients of her routine, she replied, "I do. I know when patients are in pain, I have to go down the hall to get their meds and then back up the hall to bring [them] back. That time frame is so long to them. So I do; I try to make a point of letting my patient know that I am taking a little longer, and I will be in as soon as I can. This is how I show care. I am considering their feelings." Nurses who were professionally intimate with their patients took time to tell them of any deviations in their routine or "plan for the night." They told patients when they were having a busy shift and apologized for not seeing them sooner. This demonstrated their concern for each patient and prevented patients from feeling neglected. They rushed to meet their patients' needs, and when they were delayed, they apologized and sympathized with their patients' need for them to be "on time." They knew that seeing their work from their patients' perspectives would help patients get better, because patients would feel safe and less stressed. They also knew that it was impossible to meet every patient's needs all the time; therefore, they incorporated this accountability to their patients as part of their work.

Angie, an experienced nurse, described the relationships among trust, time, and healing:

> And when they call me, I really try to get there as soon as I can be-cause I don't want to lose their trust. By the afternoon, if I don't come quickly, they'll say, "Oh, how come she doesn't come? She said she'd come." I try to keep my promise to my patients. And I find that it is this trust. The patients know that when they call me—when they want to go back to bed, they call me, and I'll be right there, or I'll send someone right there. And that trust, that really helps. If nobody came, they wouldn't want to get up out of bed again.

Angie knew that healing required her patients to become ambulatory. Ne-gotiating their movement required her to create a pact with or "promise" to patients. Whether patients would move after a painful experience depended on whether or not they trusted their nurses. Nurses knew that because pa-tients depended on them, patients needed to believe them, and they needed to believe *in* them. Experienced nurses, like Angie, learned that trust is fluid. Trust contributed to the speed and ease of healing and nurses could lose or gain their patients' trust at any time.

Many patients made comments about their nurses or asked them personal questions during the course of their hospital stay. Nurses knew that patients felt vulnerable and kept this in mind when they were asked about their private, personal lives. Patients and family members commented on nurses' choices of uniform, earrings, or hairstyle. They asked questions ranging from benign to extremely personal: about nurses' illnesses, their married lives, and their children. Nurses responded to these questions in a variety of ways. Some nurses provided brief answers, some ignored the question and redirected the conversation, and some disclosed quite a bit of information about themselves. Nurses who had experiences in common with patients disclosed more information about themselves than if their views or experiences differed from those of patients. Nurses knew that disclosing information about themselves to make them seem similar to patients was one way to connect with patients, build trust, and help them feel at ease. Nadine provided an example: "If I notice that they [my patients] were in the military, I will share that my dad was in the military." Disclosing personal and family information was something that nurses chose to do because it proved to increase patients' comfort and trust. No one explicitly instructed these nurses to disclose personal information; they discovered that introducing this kind of intimacy would help relax their patients so that they could be in a better emotional position to receive care. At the same time, recall Jody's concern earlier. Nurses had to determine—usually alone and on an individual case basis—how to negotiate the amount of personal disclosure they offered to their patients.

Nurses also negotiated intimacy with family members of patients because they believed it increased the comfort level of patients during their hospital stay. I asked nurses how they worked with families to ensure quality care. Rather than identify their own strategies, many referred me to the hospital's patient advocacy program (PAL) that institutionally permitted family members to help meet their patient's care needs during the course of a hospital stay. Jason explained how he worked with families under PAL: "With the PAL program I believe we tell them, 'This is what you're able to do. You can go get linen; you can get water.' And basically tell them they're welcome to do this but letting them know that we're also more than willing to do it. We give them options and let them choose."

Although including families in direct care contributed to healing, nurses rarely had extra time to assess whether families wanted to participate in direct care or time to demonstrate the specific care routines they used during illness and injury or monitor family involvement. Chrissy explained, "If the family member is willing to do it, then we have to show them how. If it's back surgery, we'll teach them proper routine so they don't injure themselves or the patient. Then we watch them to be sure we're comfortable that they are doing it right." Josie expressed frustration because "it's so hard to find the time. I don't know when I will do a specific thing with a patient, and then I have to make sure that the family's going to be there. If they're there, yeah, I tell them [what I'm doing]. But do I go out of my way to find them and make sure they're a part of it? No. I just don't have the time."

The program likely helped ensure quality care and patient satisfaction because it involved families in care, which seemed to increase their trust of the health-care process. It did not, however, ease the amount of labor for nurses. Although hospital administrators and family members may have thought that they relieved some of the nurses' work when they participated in PAL, the program itself actually increased the amount of nurse's work. As Jason, Chrissy, and Josie explained, nurses needed to negotiate with family members how and when they participated in patient care. In a sense, nurses were supervising family members, because it was the nurse who was institutionally accountable for the quality health care of the patient.

Although family members may want to participate in PAL (as I myself have wanted to do in similar programs in other hospitals), it does not mean that they are the most suitable caregivers for their loved one while he or she is in the hospital. Let me be clear: I do think that family members have a unique connection to their ill or injured loved one that could facilitate the intimacy needed for care (unless there is conflict between family members); however, like patients and sometimes more so, family members were fearful and stressed about the health condition of their loved one. In addition, while a patient's room might have felt like a temporary home to the patient and family, the hospital was administratively organized in such a complex way that no family member—no matter how long the hospital stay—could have accessed everything they needed to care for the patient. I observed family members, when they had questions, seeking out their nurse or waiting at the nurses' station for any available nurse to respond to them.

The PAL program was a hospital-wide project and as such was the only strategy that was systematically recognized for family care. Nonetheless, I most often observed and heard nurses describe how they worked with families outside of PAL. For example, Jill explained how her ethics of care extended to families. She described working with families by being honest and open.

I am factual, honest, ease up the mood; I just deal with families the best way that I can. I answer their questions. It's kind of like case by case. Depending on the person and what their needs are and what they want you to do for their patient. Oh definitely, I take care of them, and it's also a team. Families expect something from the doctor, the nurse. You all have to work together to get it right so that everyone is feeling comfortable.

How nurses considered families demonstrates that even their mundane intimate labor includes them. Nurses needed to ensure that patients and family members trusted them. Sometimes this need for trust could not depend on the PAL program. Nurses told me that working with families was necessary to ensure that patients received quality care, and they said that they would adjust their routines to work with families as much as they would to work with patients. Many nurses emphasized that they cared for family members as often as they cared for patients. Unlike the PAL program, this labor with families remained unnoticed.

In addition to communicating openly and honestly with family members, nurses fostered empathy for family members by imagining how they would feel if they had family in the hospital. Josie explained how and why she involved families in care: "I think they're part of the healing process for the patient. Their family's going to get them through everything. And why shouldn't they be involved? If my mother was in the hospital I would be involved in everything. So, yeah, you know, it's something I would like to do. I'm not against it in any way, unless the patient doesn't want them involved."

Similarly to how nurse administrators encouraged nurses, in their nurturing of patients, to think about how they wanted their own family members treated, experienced nurses thought about their own families when they facilitated trust with families of patients. I watched how this indeed seemed to make patients trust the care process. At the same time, however, this strategy drew on traditional expectations of femininity. That nurses explained this work as a way in which one would naturally care for family helps to sustain the idea that intimate care work is not labor, but simply activities women would want to do naturally. This keeps intimate labor hidden.

Family care complicated nurses' labor when nurses disagreed with patients' family members on how to best care for the patient. In Chapter 1, I introduce Helen, whom I had observed reassuring a patient who was dying from AIDS. The patient's family had refused hospice care, and he was nervous about going home with his parents. When she asked him why he was nervous, he told her he did not think his mother could take care of him. Recall how she said, "You are fighting [the disease] for your mom and dad, not because you have the fight in you." The patient burst into tears and said, "You are right. I do not want to do this anymore." Helen said, "I know your family refused hospice, and I don't want to step on any toes, but there are alternative programs with hospice. It doesn't mean end of life." After this conversation, the patient asked for information on counseling programs. Although Helen spent time explaining the hospice programs, detailing the outreach programs for his family, she noted in the patient's chart only that she had given a general hospice referral. There was no time to recognize the time and effort she took in counseling her patient about his options.

In addition, Helen identified and considered the family's needs in her care work, but she ultimately gave higher priority to the needs of her patient. I watched experienced nurses like Helen skillfully negotiate the needs of patients in conjunction with the needs and demands of families and doctor's orders. Helen risked losing trust with her patient to ensure that he was getting the best care. She opted for familiarity, sitting next to him on his bed and gently but firmly discussing how his family's grief and fears might be interfering with his care. Helen's care extended beyond what the nurses described as "basic care," which was just meeting the medical needs of patients. In addition to providing medical care and ensuring that her patient was physically comfortable, she assessed how and when she could approach an intimate matter—the balancing of her patient's well-being with that of his family.

Jason also explained how and when he prioritized patients' and families' needs, strategically sharing his knowledge in a way that maintained the agency of patients: "I give family choice, and I go over what I think should be done, but the patient is ultimately the boss. If it's a confused patient or a minor, it's going to be the family who makes the decision. So you can't just cut them off. But I think it's very important to give the patient choices, give them the final decision."

Even when patients were unable to make the final decision over care, Jason preserved their dignity. One way was to consider how and when he offered choices to patients, such as how to take medication (via pill or liquid). I repeatedly watched Jason simultaneously value patients and families and shift his attention accordingly to preserve each family member's agency. He maintained trust with and among all individuals.

Experienced nurses knew there were explicit relationships among trust, intimacy, and quality health care, but this knowledge and skill was virtually invisible in discourse about nursing care. Nurses worked hard to facilitate a culture of intimacy on the floor. They wanted family members and patients to feel as though they were in their homes. Nurses took care of patients and family members in private, less visible places such as in patients' rooms, behind curtains, behind closed doors, and in patients' bathrooms. They also provided care in less private areas, such as in the nurses' station and in the halls of the unit. Family members and patients roamed the units, floors, rooms, and the nurses' station to get coffee and water; put food in the refrigerator and took it out; and sat in the nurses' station to visit, process emotions, or discuss next stages of care. In all of these places, nurses were hyper-visible to patients and family members, who perceived the nurses as being accessible to them whenever they needed medical attention or intimacy. While nurses' bodies were hyper-visible, their intimate care work was hyper-*in*visible. How nurses "set the day right," chose to acknowledge or not acknowledge familiarity and personal issues, manufactured sympathy, negotiated personalities, responded to patients' inquiries, and worked with families in and mostly outside of PAL stayed off the radar.

The Social Meanings of Intimacy in Professional Care Work

Nurses noticed that race, gender, and nationality affected their negotiations of trust with their patients. How patients trusted their nurses depended on how patients perceived them according to singular categories and intersections of gender, race, and nationality. Nurses provided more or less intimate care depending on these perceptions. Women of color nurses in particular negotiated how patients and family members perceived them, to ensure trust and rapport with their patients. When I asked Bill, a white nurse, how race affected care, he talked about how whiteness informed the trust process for white patients. He said, "You know, I think the white race is the least threatening of people and that you can come across as very neutral, and I think it does help you in some respects with some people." When Bill asserted that whiteness was safe, he, by extension, implied that nurses of color are perceived as dangerous. This claim identified the relationship between race and intimate care. It also reinforced racist stereotypes because Bill did not question how whiteness has become associated with neutrality.[3] Moreover, by not specifying the race of patients and claiming that patients in general find whiteness to be least threatening, Bill generalized all patients as white. As a result, he privileged the perceptions of white patients over patients of color.

Nurses reported to me that how patients perceived professional experience was shaped in part by race and other identities. These perceptions were valuable in nursing care because patients and families used them to assess the competency of their nurses. Nurses knew that if patients perceived them as experienced, it would help those patients trust the care process. Helen, who was white and in her thirties, told me how patients assess the level of experience of nurses. She said, "I think sometimes they're trying to gauge how long you've been a nurse, so they think you're competent or know what you're doing." Tammy, an experienced white nurse in her forties, told me that she "feels bad" for young nurses who "go in there with no experience and take care of somebody twice their age." She said:

> If I was sick, I wouldn't really want a young nurse taking care of me. Well, I'd want somebody with a little experience, because there are a lot of things you can't teach people. I go in the room, and I talk, and I'm joking around with people. But you're looking at little, tiny, insignificant signs that an old nurse can pick up on and treat, and it won't become an issue, whereas a new nurse might not catch it until it's much more of a physical manifestation, more of an issue to deal with.

In their discussions of the importance of experience, most nurses across race and nationality correlated experience with age, suggesting that older age symbolically indicated more experience and younger age indicated less experience. They felt that patients perceived older-appearing nurses as experienced and younger-looking nurses as new. New nurses were instructed to mask their inexperience by appearing confident, regardless of how they felt. But Joyce, a new white nurse in her thirties, told me she did not feel insecure and that patients did not question her authority if she appeared confident. She said, "I think if you come off at the beginning as confident and in control, they do not question you because they assume you know what you're doing. They have no reason to think otherwise. If you're not sure and you're hesitant and stuff, then they have more [reason to worry]." Because I did not talk to her patients, I am not sure which combination of social identities factored into Joyce's experience of patients trusting her authority. Joyce said she just needed to "appear confident." However, the theories of whiteness and femininity I discuss in Chapter 2 suggest that Joyce's experience of patients respecting her authority as a nurse was likely constructed at the intersection of whiteness and femininity. That is, the intersection of her race and gender granted her privilege in how her patients treated her. As far as age, I am not sure. My observations of her age put her at what she identified: mid-thirties. It is possible that her patients perceived her as old enough to have cared for others and therefore experienced enough to care for them. Even if this is true, however, my analysis of age would not be uncorrupted by gender and race, because caring for others is socially feminine and not masculine and whiteness denotes professionalism. In other words, my explanation of Joyce's experience would have to include an analysis at the intersection of age, gender, and race.

My assertion that Joyce's experience was likely shaped at the intersection of whiteness and gender (and perhaps age) is strengthened when I consider my observations and interviews with women of color nurses. It was not until I spoke with nurses of color that I realized how whiteness helped inexperienced nurses look experienced and blackness and brownness detracted from perceived experience. Eva, an older-appearing and experienced African American nurse, described how a patient asked her questions about her qualifications but then automatically assumed that the white patient care technician was the nurse when Eva left the room. She told me:

> They try to get confidence in you. They will watch, and then they'll say, "How long have you been a nurse? Oh! That's why you are doing it that way. And you seem to know what you're doing." And they'll still ask you. I have some patients that I tell them I'm their nurse, and then when I leave the room, they say to the PCT, "Are you my nurse?" And the PCT is white. So that tells me that, oh, they don't think I'm the nurse. They think she is the nurse. And they start asking her questions!

Eva's experience mirrored those of several experienced, older women of color nurses who told me that patients could not see them as nurses compared to their white colleagues. Mary, an older and experienced African American nurse, explained how being African American affected her work. She said, "Sometimes when they question you regarding your training and how long you've been a nurse, they ask it in a very nice way. [*Laughs.*] They just try to ask if you are qualified." Patients consistently asked older women of color, but not white women of the same age, if they were properly trained to do nursing tasks such as listening to lungs, taking care of wounds, and administering intravenous fluids and medications.

If I stopped my analysis with age and just compared younger nurses to older nurses, it would seem that patients questioned only nurses' experience levels but not the fact that they were nurses. Instead, I learned that young, white women nurses experienced a partial rejection from patients, but women of color nurses experienced full, outright rebuff. Without an analysis of race, it seems that age is the only social identity that determines how patients perceive nurses. It is critically important to reject a color-blind rhetoric of nursing as white and feminine and just as important to reject a color-blind meaning of intimate care.

Leah, a Filipina charge nurse, also noticed that patients and family members assumed that white housekeepers, certified nursing assistants, and patient care technicians were nurses. She expressed her shock when patients and family members assumed that her white nurse assistant had more experience and education than she. She said, "For example, Ann and I—Ann is red-haired and white, and I am short, dark-haired, and Asian. I'll go into the room, and [they would see] Ann as the RN, and I would be the aide. Because how could I get my education [to be a nurse]? And there were two of us that this would happen to, and I would think, 'My God, this is a different world!'" In Leah's view, when patients and family members saw a white woman and a woman of color both entering the room to care for them, they assumed that the woman of color was less educated and therefore should have less authority than the white woman. They also assumed that the woman of color would defer to the white woman.[4] This undermined the authority of the nurse and reinforced racist ideologies that assume the superiority of and professionalization of only white people.

When I asked Carey, a new African American nurse, if patients and family members treated her differently from other nurses, she replied, "No, not really treat me differently, but they think I'm an aide. Some of them will actually grab my badge and look at it to be sure. I'll be there, close, because I'm listening to their lungs, and they'll grab my badge and look at it." Carey understood that her race affected how patients and family members perceived her. She felt the "check" of her badge reassured patients that she was their nurse and not an aide, but she still felt disrespected. Carey's anecdote illustrates how patients and family members questioned the training and qualifications of women of color nurses even while they did work that only nurses could do. Meanings of intimate care also change here. An intersectional analysis suggests that rather than tasks or demeanor, patients draw on race, gender, and nationality to identify and connect with their nurses. In my study, nurses discussed establishing and maintaining trust as one of the most important factors in ensuring quality care. Women of color nurses do not feel that their white patients trust them as easily as they do white nurses, and it is this lack of trust that alters the care exchange.

Angie, a very experienced immigrant black nurse, agreed that patients and family members assumed she was not qualified as a nurse. When she was younger, she experienced overt discrimination. Angie told me about the first time she applied for a job as a nurse. Her potential employer almost turned her away, saying the housekeeping jobs were taken. Angie said she still experienced such treatment today. Patients and family members ignored her and seemed surprised when they realized she was the nurse. Even when she introduced herself by saying, "I'll be your nurse today," patients and family members looked for someone else. She explained:

Not everybody. Some of them. I'll go in and say, "My name is so and so, and I'll be your nurse today." But then once I leave the room, the

PCT comes in, and they think she is the nurse, and they start asking her questions! The techs are nice. They are polite to say, "No I am not the nurse. The lady that just left *is* the nurse." So I'll go back in and say again that I'm the nurse and check to see if they have questions: "What kind of questions do you have?" And then they'll ask me.

Like Eva, Leah, and Mary, Angie had to repeatedly assert her professionalism to patients, despite her significant nursing experience. Leah described how a common controlling image,[5] that women of color are less educated than white women, affected how patients and family members reacted to her. Leah worried that patients who dismissed her authority would not be able to trust her competence and, therefore, would fail to trust her during intimate care. The controlling image that defined intimacy or lack of intimacy is at the intersection of race and gender because it specifies how racist and sexist ideologies construct exploitative work conditions for professional nurses of color.

The intersections of racism, sexism, and xenophobia influence not only how patients and family members identify caregivers within a particular profession but also how patients and family members understand the actual work performed by caregivers within the same profession. It is one racist-sexist-xenophobic dilemma when patients privilege the white woman as nurse and perceive the woman of color as her subordinate; it is quite another when patients misinterpret the work of nurses of color whose tasks clearly identify them as nurses. For example, one evening I followed Anna, a new Latina nurse, into her patient's room. The patient, an elderly white woman, mistakenly pressed the call light as she tried to operate her television. Anna helped her find the proper control and asked if she needed anything else. The patient pointed toward the door and said, "She's got to give it to me. I'm waiting for my pill. I'm waiting for her." Anna replied pleasantly, "What do you mean her? I am her. I am your nurse." The patient responded, "She told me she would help me." Anna reassured her patient and later brought the sleeping pills; however, her patient reacted negatively to her again. She writhed away from Anna and said, "I don't care who you are! You don't look right to me!" Anna just smiled and tried to reassure her patient. Anna told me later that when her patient said, "You don't look right to me," she thought it was because she looked and sounded Latina. She worried that her patient did not trust her because she looked like a "foreigner" and that precluded her from being someone who could safely give care. Anna not only tolerated this racist-xenophobic behavior; she also worked to help her patient overcome these attitudes so that the patient could receive intimate care.

In addition to their symbolic demotions, women nurses of color consistently field questions about their race, accent, language, and country of origin. I found in my study that sometimes, when patients responded to their nurse's race, nurses felt it was clear the patient was in fact being racist. Other times, nurses felt it was actually nationality that was in question. Sometimes race and nationality facilitated trust; other times it decreased trust. In some cases, race informed care; in others, nationality informed care. Many times interactions were constructed at the intersection of race and nationality, and sometimes interactions occurred at the intersections of race, nationality, and gender. Lydia, an Indian charge nurse, told me, "There are some times I get comments like 'Where are you from? Do you speak English? Is there anyone around here that is American and that speaks English?'" In these circumstances, patients perceive Lydia's accent as foreign, not English, and, therefore, un-American. These patients' mistrust of Lydia and sense of entitlement to an "American" nurse result from controlling images of immigration and language.

In her book *Unequal Freedom*, sociologist Evelyn Nakano Glenn explains how the social arenas of citizenship and labor have been and currently are structured by race and gender inequalities to privilege white men and subordinate women and men of color.[6] In the United States, the guarantee of full citizenship, which means full access to rights and responsibilities, ideally comes from birth, marriage, and work. Nakano Glenn's and other scholars' analyses of immigrant labor demonstrates how all of these paths to citizenship are uneven and result in unfair distributions of rights and persistent exploitations of human labor. For example, in her analysis of domestic work, Grace Chang shows how changing state legislation can dramatically affect whether or not children of immigrant workers can go to public schools.[7] Mainstream American nationalism is structured in part by anti-immigrant sentiments and manifests itself in policy that discriminates against the same people it claims to protect.[8] The socially imagined American worker is constructed against the bodies of actual workers in the United States. Anti-immigration sentiments can happen because we have a false notion of what it means to be an American worker. Nakano Glenn explains how the idea of worker citizen is constructed at the intersection of whiteness and masculinity. This is the privileged worker against which all other worker types are measured. In my research I analyze people's perceptions of nationality or citizenship by inquiring how people see skin tone, hear accents, and talk about both of these. I consider nationality as a social construct to analyze the relationship between power and interpretations of intimate care.

Mia, a Filipina nurse, explained how when patients ask her questions about her citizenship, they do so because they are uncomfortable with her accent: "When I would go into a room and I would introduce myself, and then the patient, maybe a white, older lady would say, 'Well, where are you from?' And I could see that she was uncomfortable. I felt it. They say some stuff that you know it is because of your race, because it is a trust issue."

Here, Mia is clear that race changes the experience of care because her white patients did not trust her. Moreover, she specifically marked her race as a factor in patients' mistrust when she said, "You know it is because of your race." How these patients perceived her nationality is also important to how they received or did not receive intimate care. When patients ask, "Where are you from?" it is likely in response to hearing a "foreign" accent, but it could also be in response to racialized markers like skin tone and facial features. It is not either race or nationality that affects how patients understand Mia. After considering Mia's experience, one might wonder how her gender, her age, or her sexuality might construct intimate care with patients. In other instances, there might be data that would reflect these categories. In this instance, however, it is race and nationality that are salient. This is important for conducting intersectional analyses: not all categories emerge at the same time or in the same configuration. The important thing is to notice when they do.

White nurses were less comfortable with their competence when I asked about patients of color. Nadine, a white nurse, discussed her relationships with patients of color. "I don't know how they see me. I think they might not interact with me as quickly as they would with their own race." Jody, an experienced white nurse, agreed that patients of color may have felt more comfortable with nurses of color. She said, "I wonder how much some of these black patients like us taking care of them. Quite frankly, I think they would prefer somebody within their own race."

Men and women nurses of all races contended that some complaints about bad nursing care were rooted in distrust from racist and xenophobic attitudes. Tammy and Patsy, both experienced white nurses, described how patients falsely complained to nurse supervisors as a way to refuse care from women of color. Tammy explained, "I've worked with black nurses that had patients that were really, really racist, and one patient actually wrote a letter to the nursing director. And it was totally a racist situation, but everybody knew that." Sonia, a new white nurse, described patients' relief when she entered their rooms after a Chinese nurse cared for them. She described how patients of nurses with different accents complained to her about their care. She said, "I think people do not respond as well to foreign nurses because culturally they are different." When I asked Patsy how she knew that patients' actions were racist, she replied, "They'll request another nurse. And then others will make remarks. You know, they're passive-aggressive, saying, 'She didn't do a very good job,' or 'She didn't seem to know what she was talking about.' And I know that they [nurses in question] know. But because they [nurses] have an accent, they're [patients] not willing to get the idea across to them." As Tammy's, Sonia's, and Patsy's statements illustrate, nurses noticed covert or "passive aggressive" racism and xenophobia from patients even when it did not affect them directly. Moreover, because patients are not accountable to their discomfort with racial differences, they attribute the request for a new nurse to the performance of their original nurse. If patient satisfaction forms really do, as hospital administrators claim, affect their evaluation of staff performance, then the lack of advancement by women of color nurses could be because of racist or xenophobic attitudes of patients, not the nurse's actual ability as a nurse. That all nurses who work in the United States must demonstrate standard knowledge of nursing through the required licensure and examinations, and that many countries adopted their training from U.S. models, further suggests that patients are responding from fear of cultural difference, rather than actual quality of care.[9]

Patients who inquired about the race of nurses or who outright refused nurses who were not white also demonstrate how racism shapes trust as a social interaction negotiated by intimacy. Charge nurses, team leaders, transport nurses, and other nurses who saw patients first described how patients asked about race. Roy told me, "We do have patients that are racist, 'Make sure it's not a black nurse.' Or, you know, 'Is the nurse white?' You're kind of like, 'Wow.' But if they absolutely don't want a black nurse, you got to change it. I just wouldn't know how else to—I could tell the patient that she's very good, or this and that, but if she doesn't want a black nurse touching her, then you have to make the changes." Nurses defined their professionalism in part by how they respected the beliefs of patients and family members. I observed nurses comply with racist and xenophobic requests, justifying it as an attempt to provide optimal care and to increase trust. Nurses told me that it was more practical to accommodate the patient and get someone else to take care of that patient than to argue on behalf of a nurse. This practice satisfied racist patients and likely made the nurse's life a bit easier. At the same time, these practices could contribute to the myth that women of color nurses are not professional. Moreover, these practices of switching nurses for racist patients were hyper-visible in that they were accepted practices on the unit. I noticed this visibility especially when I considered how the care of patients of color by women of color nurses was in large part *in*visible.

Black and Latina nurses felt their race and ethnicity often afforded them opportunities to care for underserved patients and family members. An African American nurse, Carey, told me she felt the presence of her darker skin tone most with Latina and black patients and family members who responded to her, pulled her into their rooms. She felt as if they brightened up when they saw her and generally seemed more relaxed in her presence. She described a situation that involved a Latino patient who reached out to her. The patient was assigned to a white, experienced nurse. He was bleeding and did not use the call light. She was down the hall on the other side of the unit when she noticed that family members sought her out. She stated:

> They kept coming out of the room looking for someone to talk to— you can tell that look. They were searching and looking. He saw me and he came over and said, "Come help us. Come help us," and I said, "No habla Española," and then one of them said, "Help my friend. Help my friend." And I knew his nurse would help, but I think they just become so distrusting. I think they look for a brown face, a friendly face, you know, "We can trust this person."

Carey told me that she knew her skin color afforded her trust with this family. Despite her not speaking Spanish or being Latina, they continued to ask her for help. Moreover, even though the charge nurse had not assigned her this family, she went out of her way to respond to them. Women nurses of color discussed how they felt called to help patients of color because they believed a nurse who "looked like them" (especially in a sea of people who did not) would make them feel more comfortable. Here, too, I analyze this circumstance of care at the intersection of nationality and race. Although Carey invoked references to nationality with her response, "No habla Española," the patients' family members appealed to her status as a woman of color, as someone who was also not white.

Mary described a special connection with an African American woman patient. "And this one lady said to me, 'Nothing against the other nurses, but you take care of me differently.' She was a black woman talking to another black woman. 'It means so much more.'" Similarly, Carey described a connection she felt with an African American diabetic patient. Nurses reported him to be "difficult" the entire two days he was on the unit because he would not talk to anybody or smile. She explained why he became more positive when she entered the room. She said, "He's trusting, because he sees someone that looks like him, and then he was scared. He was thinking they were going to cut his leg all the way up, and he felt that they didn't even care.

And a lot of older black men feel that way. They'll cut this off and cut that off, but they don't care about me as a person." In a society structured in part by racial inequalities and solidarity, trust manifested itself through perceived racial identities. The fact that this patient spoke only to Carey or that Mary's patient connected to her as another black woman exemplified that race and skin tone mattered deeply to a patient's sense of safety and security.

Language also mattered a great deal in intimate caring interactions. English-speaking nurses were concerned that Spanish-speaking patients trusted them less than they did Spanish-speaking nurses and thus were concerned that they could not provide the same care as Spanish-speaking nurses. Nadine, an English-speaking nurse, explained:

> We have a Hispanic population, and I can't speak Spanish worth crap. So a lot of times, I'll call a Spanish interpreter, and I definitely feel like it's not fair because they can't speak the language, and they don't want to ask questions. And they definitely feel more comfortable with someone of a Hispanic race. We have a tech, she goes in there, and they talk a mile a minute. When I go in there, they don't talk very much.

Nadine knew that Spanish-speaking patients interacted with her differently because she spoke only English. She regretted that her patients asked her fewer questions and spoke to her less than they did to Spanish-speaking nurses. Another English-speaking nurse, Helen, expressed concerns about language, but unlike Nadine, she admitted outright that she did not give extra care: "And if I have a Spanish-speaking patient, and the family doesn't stay at night, I can't say I don't give good care, because they will always get their medications. If they can communicate that they need something to drink or eat, they will get it. But do I go extra? No. I can't communicate with them. So they probably see me hardly at all at night."

Both nurses acknowledged that sharing the same language with your patients is critical to establishing trust. Helen distinguished between good care and going the extra mile. As a professional, she provided good care to all her patients, yet she also acknowledged that she failed to "go extra" with patients who did not speak English even though she knew that closeness and intimacy led to better care. Celia, also English-speaking, explained how she spent less time with Spanish-speaking patients. She said, "I don't speak Spanish. I don't spend as much time with them. I can't educate them, because I speak English." Like other nurses, Celia was explicit about the ways that language barriers negatively affect quality care. Simply put, speaking the patient's language increased intimate trust, which improved the quality of patient care.

Latina Spanish-speaking nurses often spoke Spanish with Spanish-speaking patients as a way to connect with them and to foster trust. Alicia, a Mexican American nurse, told me she felt a special connection with a young Mexican man new to the United States: "I went in there, and I asked if they explained to him that his toe would be amputated. And he said, 'Not really.' I told him what to expect. He asked me for my phone number. He said, 'I don't really know a lot of people here.' And I said, 'I am so sorry, I am not allowed. I could get in trouble.' He didn't understand. I honestly think he was scared. He only had his uncle."

Alicia told me that she thought perhaps this patient hoped he could see her outside of the hospital to help him build community and navigate organizations in Phoenix, which were still largely English-speaking. He likely reached out to her in part because he perceived her to be the same nationality as him in addition to the fact that she gave him special attention.

Competent, full-time, paid translators were available for nurses to use at any time at this hospital. The translation office was on the first floor of the hospital, designated to serve all medical units. Three or four translators were usually available for consult at any given time. To request a translator, nurses on each unit stopped their work to make a phone call. I witnessed nurses use a formal translator on occasion, usually for new patient intake. Typically, however, most translation needs were spontaneous, unplanned interactions. It was simply more efficient to ask nurses (and patient care technicians) who were known on the floor as Spanish speakers to stop what they were doing to perform translation. More experienced nurses who were accustomed to this routine volunteered to perform translation, but newer nurses who "looked Latina" were also asked to translate.

"Looking Latina" was reduced to skin tone. Not all Latina nurses got asked to translate immediately. Alicia, a new Latina nurse, had a pronounced Spanish accent and light skin. For two months, none of Alicia's colleagues knew that she spoke Spanish. She described a family member who thought the unit secretary spoke Spanish because she had dark skin. The family member was very surprised to learn that Alicia spoke Spanish fluently. He focused entirely on her skin tone. As she described the situation:

I'd only been there a couple of months, since October. So they are getting to know me, and a lot of them don't realize that I speak Spanish. So they call a translator, which is fine with me because I am busy with my patients, but now that they know, they go and get me. A lot of them are surprised. They say, "You speak Spanish, too?" I know I have an accent! I know I do! A family member came in and started talking

Spanish to the secretary. The secretary was dark-skinned with Spanish features but spoke absolutely no Spanish, and instead of looking at me, she started looking at her, and she was like, "I don't speak Spanish." And I said, "How can I help you?" And she said, "Oh my God! I would've thought she spoke Spanish and you were white!" And I said, "Yeah, it's funny, huh."

Alicia explained to this family member, as she later did to me, that most people assumed she was white and therefore could not speak Spanish. How her patients and her colleagues perceived Alicia was at the intersection of race and nationality. They saw her light skin and assumed she therefore would not speak Spanish. Despite the presence of Spanish-speaking white and American-born nurses, patients and family members associated Spanish with brown skin and a "foreign" accent. In this statement, Alicia also marked her parents' nationality and her ethnicity (she is first-generation Mexican American) with her accent, but others did not hear her accent. Perhaps it was trumped by her skin color. In contrast, the family member assumed the secretary (who was Native American) spoke Spanish, perhaps because she had brown skin. For both Alicia and the secretary, this family member drew on race to determine nationality.

After observing the difficulties that arose on the floor because of language barriers, Alicia began to offer her help by speaking Spanish. She soon became overwhelmed.

I get frustrated. I do. They don't pay us extra for speaking Spanish. I thought they would. They don't. When I have time, I don't mind, but [not] when I'm that busy and they don't care. For a while they would just volunteer me! Somebody would be speaking Spanish, and she [a nurse] would call me away from my work so that I could pick up the phone. I get so frustrated. Transfer the call or do something. Don't take me away from my patient. This is your job.

Latina, Spanish-speaking nurses reported mixed feelings about translation because although they liked it, they knew it was a form of exploitation. They liked translating for their colleagues because they knew that it made Spanish-speaking patients and family members feel more comfortable and increased intimate trust, which led to better care; however, it also required extra, invisible labor on an already busy shift. Although these nurses were not paid for this work, it was a form of commercialized intimacy because it contributed to quality health care and saved the hospital expense.

Anna, another new Latina nurse, was frequently asked to translate for patients and their family members. Like other Latina, Spanish-speaking nurses, Anna wanted Spanish-speaking patients because she knew it comforted them to have a Spanish-speaking nurse, but she was concerned about how often she would "get pulled" to other nurses' rooms to translate: "I get pulled a lot. And I feel that sometimes I don't get my work done, and I just have to tell them, 'Look, I'm—I'm so sorry, but I have my work to do.' And—and I just wonder sometimes, 'Why didn't they give them to me in the first place?'"

Anna's frustration was exacerbated when another nurse asked her to translate when the paid translator was already there. Her frustration lessened slightly when she realized she was communicating more successfully with the patient than the paid translator since she understood the patient's dialect and slang. She told me, "So he understood me and was asking me questions. And I don't know if the other translator was getting mad. So that's another thing. I'm pretty good at it, especially medical stuff—I'm good at it. I'm pretty good at translating."

Anna knew that she was good; in fact, she viewed herself as "one of the translators" when she referred to the possibility that the "*other*" translator might be getting angry. She identified her skill—translating difficult and complicated medical jargon into a particular Spanish dialect. Although she used this skill at work regularly, she was neither recognized nor compensated for it. Since hospitals often need immediate translation—the kind that cannot wait for a translator to be summoned from another floor—nurses like Anna were regularly expected to meet this need. The hospital garnered benefits from this form of convenient and unpaid translation, such as better and more efficient communication, increased trust, and the avoided expense of formal translators.

Conclusion

To provide quality health care, nurses negotiated intimacy in a professional manner and within specific economic constraints. Ostensibly seamless against a backdrop of economic insecurity, nurses created a safety net. When there were not enough nurses, individual nurses increased their intimate workload. When patients feared that their health insurance was not sufficient, nurses made them feel better and bureaucratically pushed to continue care. These negotiations were constant and mundane; intimacy was important not only to maintain care but also to develop trust. Nurses worked in and around "intimate settings" and with patients and family members who had "intimate ties" to each other.[10] Nurses alleviated patients' fears by building intimate trust and familiarity through consistent reassurances, addressing disclosures and biases, and balancing individual needs against a turbulent work environment. For nurses to provide intimate trust from the perspective of the patient, they needed skill, strategy, time, and practice. Moreover, although nurses identified intimacy as a critical part of nursing care, it was invisible labor. Not all new nurses knew how intimacy would be part of their work. Administrators, too, did not understand the rhythm and tone to intimate care. Institutional measures to promote inclusion and quality—PAL and formal translation—were not consistently useful to nurses. They either required nurses to do more work (as in the case of PAL) or did not serve as well as nurses did themselves (as in the case of formal translation). I found that in both cases, and although invisible to administrators, nurses developed their own strategies to nurture and provide intimate trust to patients and their families across different identities.

How patients perceived their nurses was a significant factor in how intimate trust was accomplished. For some patients, these perceptions were shaped by racism and xenophobia and needed to be analyzed with both patient care and nurse retention in mind. This hospital could lose good nursing staff if they did not start to hold patients accountable to these biases and find ways to reassure them outside of reinforcing prejudices. The first step might be to acknowledge that these prejudices and preferences informed the care process and that there was no universal predictor of or provision for intimate care. At the same time, marginalized patients—those of color and who were Spanish-speaking—gained much intimate trust from nurses of color who made them feel safe in a state (Arizona) that many perceive as unsafe and as encouraging of anti-immigrant sentiments.

I found intersectionality to be an incredibly useful approach to analyzing the value, labor, and meaning of intimate trust. In some cases, patients drew on well-established controlling images at the intersection of race and gender—for example the false universal that women of color are less educated than white women. Here, I am thinking how Eva, Leah, Mary, and Angie were consistently not identified as nurses by their patients. I explain these patients' conclusions by using Patricia Hill Collins's idea of controlling images: dominant, untrue ideologies about women of color that inform and contribute to unequal labor and other material experiences. These and other examples explain how social identities construct the process of intimate care, but here I highlight Mia's, Carey's, and Alicia's experiences as examples of intersectionality when some social identities make meanings of others. Mia talked about how trust was affected by her race, but I contend that her trust with patients could have been affected by how patients perceived her nationality, since they often asked questions about her citizenship (e.g., "Where are you from?"). Carey's Spanish-speaking patient made meaning from her race that helped him trust her. Although their nationalities differed, it was her skin color that mattered most to gain intimate trust with this patient. Alicia's patient drew from common ideologies about race to determine Alicia's language abilities. The patient thought Alicia was white because she was light-skinned and therefore that she would not be able to speak Spanish. These examples reveal how intimate trust is negotiated at intersections of race, gender, and nationality. They also demonstrate how meanings of social identities rely on each other and are not fixed. This helps disrupt the relationship between naturalness and social identity.

This first stage of professional intimacy, intimate trust, challenges dichotomous framings of nursing—that it is either professional or nurturing, labor or love, skill or nature, altruistic or paid. The concept of professional intimacy demonstrates that nursing is all these things and that professional intimacy is dialectic, reflecting a tension produced from the need for and the result of intimacy in professional work. Professional intimacy results from and affects care interactions among nurses, patients, and family members. In my study, these exchanges were affected by the intersections of race, gender, and nationality. Depending on the identities of individuals involved, these interactions both reinforce and challenge dominant ideologies that care occurs naturally, that people are either inherently caring or they are not, and that altruism is a pleasant experience. But care work in nursing is not a natural process; it requires specialized knowledge and experience. Moreover, people successfully do care work whether or not they consider themselves inherently caring individuals. Finally, at odds with common definitions of what it means to be caring and to be cared for, altruistic interactions sometimes result in conflict for the patient and for the nurse.

4

Slurs, Pickup Lines, and Intimate Conflicts

When I began to discuss with nurses how they negotiate conflict with patients, many talked about conflict that happens on the "psych" floor, in the "psych" unit, or with "psych" patients. When I designed my study, I purposefully avoided the psychiatric unit, the emergency room, or other units that had already been identified as units with "difficult" patients or unusual circumstances. Nonetheless, I found that the reputations of these units and these patients traveled to the units I studied. That is, there existed a dominant idea that the potentially violent patients or the "difficult" patients existed elsewhere in the hospital. The nurses I studied were not prepared for, nor did they think they would need to manage, conflict from their patients, because they worked with "general patient" populations. When new nurses discussed conflict they talked about being surprised; when experienced nurses talked about it, they said it did not happen often. While this was true for individual nurses, I observed a significant pattern of intimate conflict that happened normally as part of establishing trust through intimate care. I submit that nurses do not see intimate conflict as readily as I did because (1) they are focused on their own individual practice and not trained to think in collective terms, (2) they are trained to identify and negotiate conflict only in specialized populations, and (3) universal meanings of care do not include conflict or money (instead, care is defined as natural, moral, and sacred).

In general, professional labor is defined through maintaining emotional, physical, and sexual boundaries. For example, formal policies exist that prohibit physical and sexual interactions in professional work. Professional workers also maintain boundaries at work by caring for clients publicly while keeping their own emotions private. In nursing, however, nurses encourage familiarity and trust with their patients to help them receive quality health care. In Chapter 3, I show how nurses establishing intimate trust with patients relax nurse-patient boundaries. In this chapter, I describe how these relaxed boundaries are emotional, physical, and sexual and can cause conflict for the nurse. I argue that intimate conflict will happen with patients regardless of the illness and injury they suffer. This conflict occurs in the context of commercialized intimacy because it occurs as a market exchange: patients pay and hospitals profit.

I establish that intimate conflict is a part of professional intimacy because patients develop familiarity with nurses, which might enable them to express their needs and concerns more readily. This increased sense of familiarity may help patients to feel entitled to constant care from their nurses. How patients feel entitled to care is likely exacerbated by a health-care system that focuses on profits rather than needs. Because health care is defined by capital and patients are increasingly defined as consumers, hospitals feel increasingly obligated to provide an environment that offers service. Patients may also be more likely to feel entitled to service that one might receive in other types of service industries. On the other hand, patients may feel entitled to the care they receive because they rarely feel cared for in a system dominated by the interests of health management organizations. I observed how relaxed boundaries and a sense of entitlement sometimes encouraged patients to express anger and sexual desire toward their nurses. As a result, nurses felt and negotiated discomfort, tension, and harm to sustain intimate trust.

Entitlement to Service

A general conflation of care with service contributed to patients' feelings of entitlement to constant satisfaction and comfort. On patient satisfaction reports, patients said that special and extra food and drink, extra blankets, extra attention, and other acts of service by nurses were acts of caring. They acknowledged these acts of service more than they did medical care or technical expertise. Nurses told me that some patients expected them to meet these needs in part because patients developed a sense of familiarity and trust with their nurses. Other nurses suggested that patients might demand service because this was all they could control about their stressful hospital stay. Mostly, however, nurses told me that patients misunderstood their jobs and thought that service was part of nursing.

Nurses had a different perspective. Although nurses did not count service in their scope of care practice, they provided service because their patients valued these acts as good care. Many nurses asserted that providing service to patients was central to good care because patients expected service—the kind of service one might expect in a hotel or restaurant—while in the hospital. Nurses also knew that these simple acts, such as giving warm blankets, made patients feel special and safe. It was these simple acts of service that helped to build intimacy and maintain trust. This resulted in a vicious cycle. Patients' senses of entitlement to service increased as their nurses responded to them. When patients did not feel satisfied by nursing care, they could become frustrated, which sometimes caused conflict for the nurse.

Patients sometimes expressed feelings of entitlement and frustration through verbal and physical confrontation to make sure their needs were met. Jane, an experienced nurse, expected this kind of conflict from patients: "I think it is part of their care. You never know why patients act the way they act. You know, sometimes it can be something emotionally, and sometimes they can be ruder. I don't mind, because I think it's a need. I think they feel they need to have the hospital satisfy how they feel." Although experienced nurses told me that conflict with their patients was rare, they also said that they assumed that patients would feel entitled to extra attention from them and would react negatively if they did not get it. Over time, nurses learned to take responsibility for these confrontations and include them in their care of patients. It would seem, then, that handling conflict would be considered a normal part of nursing care. However, because it remained unarticulated in collective discourse, this labor went unnoticed. Therefore, although experienced nurses would care for patients by meeting their needs for service, privately they felt disrespected and frustrated when patients expressed needs or sentiments they considered inappropriate or excessive.

Some nurses expressed discomfort with what they felt was an expression of excessive and inappropriate gratitude from patients. For example, patients and family members often gave nurses gifts like food, candy, and stuffed animals to thank them for their hospital experience. Some patients even offered extra money or "tips" to nurses for good care. Jody explained, "They just appreciate their care, and they want to express it, but, you know, we already get paid. [*Laughs.*]" Although nurses knew that patients intended to show gratitude, nurses felt that patients who offered gifts and tips recognized the relationships produced from intimate care rather than the professional skill that was required to produce these relationships. Moreover, the act of giving a tip symbolizes work that is service-oriented; the act of giving a gift mirrors a personal relationship. Neither act acknowledges professional labor. These acts highlight commercialized intimacy in nurse-patient relationships.

Nurses also expressed discomfort with patients who made requests that to them seemed beyond the scope of quality care. Depending on their circumstances, patients felt entitled to additional food, a longer stay in the hospital, increased medication, and increased attention. For example, patients sometimes complained about food preferences or the timing of their medications. At the beginning of each day, dietary staff would come into each patient's room and help him or her choose their food for each meal. Sometimes after patients received the meals, they complained to nurses, "Well, I didn't order this" and asked questions such as "Well, what's this?" or "Can you get me skim milk?" Or they said, "I want apple juice, not orange juice" or "This is too hot. This is too cold." Amy, an experienced nurse, explained, "If patients didn't get exactly what they wanted, or if it was hot or cold or whatever, all they had to do was call the nurse, and you just kind of got the brunt of it." Patients saw dietary staff once a day, but nurses were always on the floor, within reach. Patients did not have a trusting relationship with dietary staff, but they did with their nurses. They knew that nurses were accessible, and they felt comfortable going to them first. Nurses had to field complaints and concerns outside of their scope of practice and sometimes resented patients and family members who they felt manipulated them to get what they wanted. When nurses perceived that patients had an unfair sense of entitlement to service, they became frustrated. Amy clarified: "I don't like rude family members, demanding patients, patients who treat you as if you are a waitress or their housekeeper. It's the tone of voice that they have. And then you have six patients—blood transfusions, this one needs pain medicine, you need to start an IV over here. I mean, you've got other stuff going on that is much more a priority than juice." Nurses became frustrated when their professional labor was reduced to service, but they also reacted to the circumstances of their labor, which resulted in a constant time crunch—too much work to do in too little time. Nurses felt devalued when patients focused on service rather than their professional and medical expertise and became increasingly and understandably frustrated when they felt simultaneously devalued and overworked.

Nurses talked about how patients also expected them to serve their families. Leah described feeling conflicted about a patient who expected the hospital to pay for her husband's meals:

One month ago, an American Indian who lived up north was transferred here because there was no hospital where she lived. Her husband had no place to stay, so he stayed in the room with his wife. And she expected us to feed her husband. He didn't have any money or any place to go. See, we were caring for the patient and not the husband. But she expected us to serve the husband. When I was working one day, she asked me if I could get her husband something to eat. I just said "I—we have a cafeteria. He can go downstairs and get some food, but I cannot give him a tray." But then I said, "What I can do is give him an extra tray if no one needs it, but I can't give him a tray every meal." Patients expect their family to be fed at the same time as them. And you just have to get the boundary there. We will care for you, but we can't care for your family.

In the beginning and the end of her commentary, Leah said that service was not part of nursing. However, Leah also said she had offered to get a plate for her patient's spouse if an extra tray was available. Even though Leah and other nurses insisted that service was not in their scope of practice, they still practiced service to try to best meet the needs of their patients. In this sense, nurses negotiated requests for service as part of professional intimacy.

Nurses negotiated requests for service, but they also felt that their efforts were taken for granted. When I asked Josie, a newer nurse, if service was part of care, she said:

I do service. But does the patient know I have so many things to do that are more important? I think I've said, "I'm not a waitress. This isn't the Hilton." I need to make sure they're drinking, but do I need to make sure that they have the exact drink that they want and they desire on the floor at all times? I have to go out of my way to call dietary and make sure this drink comes up. Or I've gone down to a pop machine because they just insisted on a Diet Sprite.

Like Amy and Leah, Josie felt tension between providing service to patients and resenting patients for requests that seemed unreasonable. Josie knew that meeting patients' requests for a particular food or drink extended outside her scope of practice, a practice that was already overburdened with paperwork, coordination activities, and care. She tried to meet these needs, however, because she, like most nurses, knew how patients valued this attention, so she strategically incorporated meeting these requests into her routine.

Although nurses were willing to serve patients, it was more difficult for nurses to alter their routine when patients were dishonest with them. Chrissy, a new nurse, felt betrayed when she discovered a patient had lied to her about his food: "The way he was telling me, he was complaining of the food being so bad. We ordered another tray, and he ate the first tray. Why in every meal [would you] complain about food and then eat both of them? At first you feel for them and you believe. Order another tray and another tray. And I realized then that he was lying all along. I said, 'God, he is manipulative.'"

Chrissy believed her patient when he complained that his food was spoiled, but soon realized that he was lying to her so that he could get more meals. She was frustrated because he wasted her time and the time of other staff members, but more so, because she needed him to honestly express his needs so that she could best do her job. Nurses depended on their patients to honestly communicate their needs. When they failed to communicate honestly, patients interrupted the potential for optimal professional intimacy and needlessly overworked their nurses.

Nurses' feelings of disrespect were aggravated when patients seemed impossible to satisfy. Celia, a newer nurse, explained that some patients and family members expected constant attention but were never satisfied: "The rude ones—overtly rude—who are overtly demanding; the ones who call every five minutes, and no matter what you do, you're not going to make them happy; the family who thinks my whole purpose is to take care of their mom. You spend all of your time on this patient [so] that all the rest get neglected."

Leah also described demanding patients as those who "can't be pleased." Demanding patients and family members treated nurses "rudely" and "unreasonably." They treated nurses with disrespect and acted entitled to them. Demanding patients could quickly turn into abusive patients. Lydia explained this fine line:

> No nurse has to be in an abusive situation. We have patients who are coming off the drugs, and they get very hungry. And they'll say, "I want a steak and potatoes," and the best we can do is get a hamburger and fries. And one patient was eating so much ice cream that she emptied our supply for the whole night. And then when I told her that I didn't have any, she told me I was lying and that I was being rude. It got so bad that my nurses could not continue their work.

Depending on the patient and the circumstances, the simplest requests could escalate to abusive or unfair treatment. Both patients and nurses could conflate service and care. In part from the familiarity and trust they gained from establishing trust in professional intimacy, patients felt entitled to good service. Nurses distinguished entitled patients from needy patients by describing entitled patients as "difficult," demanding, and disrespectful to them. Nurses expected patients to need. Needy patients asked questions, expressed pain, pressed the call light, and wanted to talk. Moreover, because professional intimacy is an exchange, in order to do their jobs nurses *needed* patients to express their needs. Most nurses felt that providing service to patients was part of care, although some found it annoying. All patients were needy patients, but entitled patients, nurses said, "acted out." When entitled patients felt frustrated or expressed pain, stress, or fear, they could become angry and hurtful.

Types of Conflict

Nurses experienced angry patients and family members as part of professional intimacy, but conflict also resulted from establishing intimate trust. Not all patients became angry and abusive to alleviate fear and feelings of powerlessness, but when they did, two patterns emerged: patients expressed either inappropriate anger or inappropriate sexual behaviors (desire or interactions). Although each nurse told me that she or he rarely experienced violent or sexual behaviors from patients, I observed patterns of patients sexually interacting with nurses and with guests, patients stepping outside of their rooms and demanding nurses for attention, patients shoving or kicking nurses, and patients and family members yelling at nurses out of pain or frustration.

Angry and Abusive Interactions

Patients exploited and abused nurses to alleviate their feelings of fear and powerlessness. While some of these interactions resulted from drug and alcohol detoxification or involved patients who were mentally unstable, many resulted from ordinary patients who felt pain, stress, fear, and entitlement. These interactions included extreme violence, such as yelling at nurses, grabbing them forcefully, and threatening to harm them. Brett asserted, "We as nurses take a lot of abuse in general. Just, actually two nights ago, a male patient came out of the room screaming and yelling at his nurse. He walked up to the nurses' station and was very vocal, using abusive language." Eva also said, "They holler, scream, and they're scared. They're scared. They're really scared, you know." Nurses "took abuse" because they understood that patients and family members expressed anger out of fear, pain, and frustration.

Part of nurses' intimate labor was to reduce intimate conflict, because these interactions affected how nurses could care for patients. A patient's anger directed at a nurse especially stifled possibilities for intimate trust.

Moreover, intersections of gender, race, and nationality structured intimate conflicts as they did intimate trust. Jackie, a Filipina new nurse said, "They have anger; [they get] frustrated, sad, and that can affect how they treat you and react to you." She described an interaction with a white man who became very agitated, making racist and xenophobic remarks when she asked him where he would like his IV for his pain medication.

> Then he just got so upset, and then he called his daughter saying, "Take me home now." He moved his arm, and I realized it was a pick line [permanent IV for medication]. I gave him the medication, and then I said, "Do you have anything you want to tell me?" He said, "I want my daughter to send me to a hospital with only white people." And I said, "Why?" And he said because "I cannot trust a person who doesn't even understand English." And I say, "I understand English."

Jackie's patient focused his fear and anxiety about his illness on his fear of Jackie's nationality, accent, and language. He felt entitled to a hospital that had only white people and a nurse that spoke only English. Language—as a marker of nationality—informed the meaning of race for this patient. This intersection of race and nationality informed his meaning of nursing care. Moreover, although Jackie spoke English, her patient constructed her as non-English-speaking. This construction was also at the intersection of race, gender, and nationality. The patient could have reacted to Jackie's skin tone, facial features, accent, femininity, or a combination of any of these things. These social identities cannot be analyzed separately.

Women of color nurses tolerated abuses from patients reacting to race, gender, or nationality, but this did not mean that they consented to these behaviors. Instead, they hoped to care for their patients as well as they could and often internalized their patients' perceptions of them. Jackie suggested that "patients don't like me just because I am an Oriental girl." When she told me this, she slightly shrugged her shoulders as if to say there was nothing she could do—slurs were a burden she must bear. Jackie and other nurses had no recourse against these slurs, because intimate conflict is not recognized as an established part of nursing care. Intimate conflict is discussed in natural, unpredictable terms in part because intimate care is defined as a natural trait that cannot be socially regulated or changed.

Slurs and other expressions of anger changed the process of intimate care. In some cases nursing care under these conditions is halted, and in other cases nurses do additional and invisible work to negotiate care. Although Jackie and other nurses of color told me they tolerated these abuses to maintain professionalism, remarks by these patients undermined intimate trust and familiarity. Mary, an experienced African American nurse I introduced previously, described a patient who drew on a familiar, racist-sexist controlling image—the mammy—to feel comfortable with her:[1] "Since I am an African American, I remember very vividly the one patient who told me that I was like his mammy that used to care for him. He was an older gentleman. I think he was feeling cared for. I'm like, 'Please not while I am cleaning you up!' But he was feeling cared for. As an African American, black woman, did he feel like I would take offense? I don't know."

I discuss this incident in Chapter 2 as a way to help explain the power of controlling images to normalize inequalities.[2] Mary's example with her patient also illustrates how intersections of race and gender change the meaning of doing care work. Mary told me she felt subservient and "like a slave" to her patient, but she tolerated these feelings and stifled her discomfort. She chose to mask her uneasiness because she knew that open acknowledgment of his understanding of the intersection of her race and gender would increase his comfort and increase her professionalism. However, this tolerance and negation of intimate conflict did not happen easily. It was extra, unrecognized labor that she had to perform to maintain intimate trust with her patient.

Nurses told me that, many times, patients expressed anger because they did not understand their illness or their treatment and felt scared and powerless. Nurses simultaneously empathized with patients' feelings of powerlessness and endured unfair treatment from these same patients. Mary explained that "patients tend to get angry" when they get conflicting information about their care. Nurses in my study thought that patients rightly expected consistent information from their health-care providers. They understood the frustration of patients when their nurses were limited in how much information they could provide. Mary explained, "Like if a patient has a couple of physicians on the case telling him conflicting information, and they look to the nurse to clarify the situation. As a nurse I think you feel limited in your powers and how much you can say because you don't always have the okay." This "okay" referred to the physician's decision about care as well as the approval to share information with the patient.

Nurses were more likely to tolerate difficult, even violent, interactions if they thought their patients felt particularly vulnerable or scared, rather than if they thought their patients felt entitled to service or attention. Trixie understood that the anger and abuse came from her patient feeling intense pain and hunger, not from his feeling entitled to service or a personal connection to her. She explained how she endured her patient's abuse: "You don't yell at them back. And you have to understand that this person hasn't eaten for hours and hours and hours. He was told his surgery was going to be at this time [and now it is delayed]. So I think, put myself in his shoes; but still it's hard because it's hard not to take it personal."

Trixie empathized with her patient as a way to tolerate the abuse. In nursing school, students are taught to empathize with patients and to see care from the patient's perspective, but they are not necessarily taught how to manage these behaviors or see how they are connected to intimate trust. Just because Trixie understood her patient's pain and hunger did not mean that she felt no discomfort in return. Although Trixie knew not to take her patient's behaviors personally, she acknowledged that it was still difficult.

Nurses empathized with their patients, but they too endured pain and abuse as a result of how patients coped with their pain. Lori, a new nurse, discussed a patient who in extreme pain tightly squeezed her hand to the point that she too felt physical pain. When she asked him to stop, he coped with his pain by hitting and kicking another nurse who was also caring for him at that time. Lori explained: "One patient had my hand really tight, and I would tell him, 'Let go of my hand. You're hurting me. Let go of my hand.' And after, you know, kind of negotiating—well not negotiating—but after a few minutes he would let go of my hand, but then he would start hitting and kicking and trying to do something to the other person who was there help-ing me. So, I don't confront it if I don't have to."

Lori assessed that her patient could not control himself when the patient tried to stop hurting her hand and then kicked and hit another nurse. She did not confront this patient because she knew that he was coping with his pain through physical reaction and that if he was not hurting her, he would likely hurt another staff member. Instead, she does "not confront if I don't have to." Lori's experience extends the idea of simply tolerating abuse to maintain intimacy essential to conducting emotional and body labor.

In her book *The Managed Hand: Race, Gender, and the Body in Beauty Service Work*, sociologist Miliann Kang extends Arlie Hochschild's concept of emotional labor. Kang coins and conceptualizes body labor, the commercial-ization of bodies in service work. She writes:

> The term body labor designates commercialized exchanges in which service workers attend to the physical comfort and appearance of the customers, through direct contact with the body and attending to the feelings involved in these practices. . . . I use body work as a general term for referring to commercial and non-commercial efforts

directed at maintaining and improving the health and/or appearance of the body.[3]

Kang theorizes body labor across intersections of race, gender, and citizenship to capture how bodily contact between workers and consumers is not monolithic but operates at the intersection of various social identities. Body labor helps us examine how the bodies of workers and consumers reinforce social inequalities—how some bodies are made normative (i.e., white hospital patients) and some bodies are socially subordinate. Emotional labor emphasizes the management of commercial feelings; body labor focuses on the management of embodied exchanges. Nurses may employ body labor, like emotional labor, to maintain professional intimacy. Lori conducted body and emotional labor because this work contributed to the patient's health care and satisfaction, but it was not recognized by anyone else other than Lori. If we think about how nurses conduct emotional labor and body labor as part of their work in the hospital, we can imagine how over time the hospital financially benefits from these forms of commercialized intimacy because this labor is expected as part of patient satisfaction and naturalized as part of nurse work.

Nurses knew that some patients could not control their actions and acted in response to physical pain or mental disorientation. They believed that these patients did not react out of entitlement, but rather out of confusion. They distinguished these patients from those who purposefully reacted violently out of frustration or feelings of entitlement. As Mia explained, "Patients who would try to hurt you, they're mad at you, they could throw a pitcher of water at you. There was a patient that came in and he had a knife there. He started to get the knife and he was going to stab me because he was so mad about the situation." Mia thought that this patient reacted violently not because he was feeling physical pain or fear, but because he was "mad." Other nurses described patients who verbally or physically threatened them. For example, Amy described a patient who walked off the unit and locked himself in another room. Amy and another nurse followed the patient and asked him to unlock the door. When he did, he became extremely violent when she and the other nurse approached. Amy explained, "My colleague said to the patient, 'Let's go back to your room.' She put her hand to, you know, to walk, and he goes like he's going to take her hand, and he just gets his arm, and he just gets her around the neck, like in a choke hold. And so, I was grabbing his arm to pull him off, and then he came after me, and he, like, grabbed me by the hair and threw me on the ground."

I asked Amy how the hospital reacted to her physical assault. She told me that she took personal leave, and the CEO sent her flowers. Thankfully,

Amy did not experience serious injuries, but she did experience trauma. As a professional, Amy handled this conflict on her own by taking some time off from work to recover. She also told me she thought there was nothing else that could have been done. Amy might have felt differently if she had known her experience was not an isolated one.

Helen described a patient who threatened to kill another nurse because the nurse had not retrieved his medication from the pharmacy quickly enough. The frustrated patient called down to the pharmacy, and the pharmacy contacted the hospital nurse supervisor to address the problem. When the nurse supervisor arrived on the floor, he rushed past the nurse and went directly to the patient. After seeing the patient, the supervisor reprimanded the nurse for not medicating the patient quickly. Helen explained that she was upset with the nurse supervisor because he did not address the patient's threat.

> This was no empty threat, as he [the patient] had hit another doctor in the hospital. The threat was there. I agree, we just have to give him his meds, but the patient had not listened to his nurse. She couldn't get in touch with pharmacy. The nurse supervisor never addressed the issue with the patient—that he can't talk to staff that way. That's a threat. Anywhere else, the supervisor would have called the cops. There is no policy in place, no repercussions for patients if they threaten a nurse.

There was no institutional protection from potential verbal or physical harm from patients because the hospital did not think that these incidents normally occurred. The hospital did not acknowledge these encounters until after they occurred, and when they did, they either blamed individual nurses or thanked them for handling the conflict. As a result, floor and charge nurses addressed angry patients with little if any institutional support.

Nurses tolerated angry and abusive slurs from patients that came from entitlement, fear, and racism-sexism-xenophobia. They negotiated these interactions to maintain professional intimacy, whether or not they felt patients were acting manipulatively. They felt empathy for the patient, whether or not they thought patients had control over their actions. Although they disliked these situations, nurses tried not to take them personally but instead aimed for patient satisfaction because this is what they believed would lead to quality care. Nurses skillfully addressed intimate conflict alone or with one or two other colleagues. They received no institutional support or recourse when patients acted out. The skillful emotional and body labor they used to regain intimate trust with their patients was invisible.

Sexualized Interactions

In addition to experiencing verbal and physical harassment, nurses encountered a wide range of sexualized interactions and situations from patients and family members. These ranged from harmless flirting to more intense physical touch and requests for sexual stimulation. Patients flirted with nurses and made comments about their bodies and appearance. Patients also persistently taunted, leered at, and physically touched nurses. They propositioned nurses and requested sexual stimulation. They tried to kiss nurses and grabbed their buttocks and breasts. Even nurses who did not personally experience sexual interactions involving patients and family members described incidents that happened to other nurses. Moreover, nurses were forced to deal with patients who, during their hospital stay, were intimate with their visitors in ways that included hugging, kissing, sleeping in the same bed, and engaging in sexual intercourse.

Sexual Interactions Involving Patients

Sexual interactions involving patients did not just cause conflict for the individual nurse; they also challenged the idea that professional care is inherently nonsexual. In the beginning of each interview or informal conversation, most nurses told me they "rarely" experienced sexual interactions involving patients and family members. Later in our talks, however, each nurse described at least one story of sexualized interaction. Here, I suggest that part of what makes sexualized interactions both pervasive and invisible in nursing care is how they are discussed as natural and inevitable interactions. Instead of seeing patients as both being dependent and having agency over their own behaviors, many nurses remarked that patients were too dependent to sexualize their hospital stay.[4] If patients could not control themselves because they were dependent, negotiating sexual interactions involving them became inevitable and did not need to be discussed as a workplace issue. The problem here is that it is possible for an individual to be dependent on another person and choose to not sexually interact with that person, which means that patients could choose to not be sexually inappropriate with nurses. Nurses also explained sexualized behaviors by saying they were from patients who were confused and, thus, unaware of their behaviors, but from my observations, I know that not all patients who engaged with nurses sexually were confused. Some older nurses thought that patients might sexualize younger nurses but would not find interest in them. This explanation limits sexual interactions in the workplace as having sexual interest in colleagues and not as a site to negotiate power. There is a difference between having sexual interest in someone and being sexually inappropriate. Patients do not have to have sexual interest in nurses to use sexuality as a means to gain power. Nurses felt discomfort from patients who were sexual, but they negated or justified sexual conflict by seeing patients as dependent, confused, or having harmless sexual interest.

Although many nurses did not define sexualized interactions from patients and family members as sexual harassment, these interactions disrupted professional intimacy and the potential for optimal care. Josie did not think sexualized interactions were sexual harassment but said they affected how she cared for patients: "But as much as I don't define it as sexual harassment, does it affect my caring for that patient? Yeah, because I'll ignore [the patient]; I will not go into that room as much. Or I'll ignore him more than my other patients. I won't want to deal with it." Danae also asserted, "Somebody told one of the nurses that she had a nice, nice ass, you know. That he liked to watch, watch her come in the room. You know, and that, right there, now the nurse doesn't want to go in there anymore." Nurses knew that how patients interacted with them affected care. If nurses did not know how to professionally negotiate these kinds of intimacies, patient care suffered.

Young and new nurses expressed surprise over the frequency of sexualized comments and behaviors from patients and family members. Josie told me that she heard a sexualized remark, usually from a younger man, at least once a day. Joyce, a new nurse in her thirties, described an inappropriate comment from a patient. She said, "It was this old guy, and he was paralyzed. And he just made all these comments like 'I need a back rub. You have a nice ass, even though you're a little thick. Your husband must treat you good because you're always smiling.'" She grimaced. "He meant good in bed." As with the slurs previously described in this chapter, new nurses felt discomfort when men patients sexualized them, but they tolerated these pickup lines from patients to maintain a combination of professionalism and intimate trust. They tolerated them because they did not know what else to do.

Nurses also described male patients who simultaneously exposed themselves and propositioned their nurses. Josie said that patients did this "a lot. They'll basically ask to sleep with you. It's gotten to the point where there are male patients who will literally just lift their clothes up and hang out and talk about their size and stuff." Josie knew that patients were deliberate in their exposures because they combined these actions with verbal requests for sex and descriptions of their sexual prowess. Patients also propositioned nurses in front of their spouses. Sonia described a patient whose "wife was sitting in there and he said something totally inappropriate, especially in front of her, like, 'What are you doing later?' or 'You could come home with me.'" Patients simultaneously sexualized nurses and did not consider how these interactions would affect their spouses or the nurses. They both did the act and minimized the act. They could minimize the act in part because they did not consider nurses to be legitimate social actors in these exchanges. The purpose of the nurse in their minds was to care for the patient and meet the patient's needs. The dichotomous view that nurses are either sexy or maternal exacerbates the negation of nurses' agency.[5] As Bridget Anderson describes, both care work and the bodies that do this care work are commodified.[6] Patients rightly felt entitled to good care, but sometimes this sense of entitlement extended to nurses as well.

Male nurses also described how men and women patients made sexualized remarks about their appearance. For example, Bill explained how gay men patients or visitors commented on his looks. He said, "I've taken care of a few gay men patients that have mentioned to their partner, 'Did you see my nurse today? He's really cute.' You know, and things like that. And I usually don't respond back to that." Jason discussed his discomfort when men patients propositioned him. He explained one case: "He was kind of making suggestive coming-on comments. And I was not comfortable, but I mean, I didn't shun him. I wouldn't consider it [sexual harassment] because it was not overt." Brett also experienced propositions from men patients. Although he was not uncomfortable, he thought these interactions were inappropriate. He said to patients, "That's inappropriate. I'm your nurse. I'm here to take care of you." He told me that he simply tells patients, "Comments like that will not be tolerated." Jason ignored these behaviors because he did not want to make them worse. Bill did not think they merited attention. In contrast, Brett described why he confronted sexualized behaviors from patients immediately. He said, "I felt really degraded, personally as well as professionally."

In the first month of my study, I observed Jackie try to manage the sexual advances of an older, white man during her care for him. When she helped him back to bed, he grabbed her arms, grabbed her shirt, and asked her to come to bed with him. She later told me that he grabbed her breasts. I heard her say, "Hey, what are you doing? I am not your wife!" I watched her leave his room and quickly move to her next patient's room. It seemed that she had no time to reflect on the exchange between her and her patient. When she had a free moment, I asked her about the interaction. She told me her patient was "confused" and disoriented because of his medication.

Two days later in the staff room, Jackie told me that the same patient was sitting in a regular chair in the nurses' station "visiting" the nurses. When Jackie walked by him, he abruptly grabbed her from behind and pulled her down on his lap. I asked Jackie if she thought this was part of her job. She exclaimed in shock, "What? To sit on his lap? Of course not!" When I asked her why she did it, she seemed unsure. Although initially Jackie seemed uncomfortable with my questions, she later told me that the patient "wasn't too bad," and she knew "he liked me." I asked her how she knew this, and she did not say; she just shrugged her shoulders.

When Jackie left the staff room, Mimi, an experienced patient care technician who had listened to the conversation, said, "They need to be told." I asked, "By whom?" She said, "By the person who they do that to." Mimi told me the majority of patients who "cross the line" stop when they are told to do so. She agreed that educators do not teach nurses how to stop inappropriate behavior, but that nurses learn how to do this over time. She said, "The girls should be trained because some men are just like that." I asked Mimi how nurses should stop inappropriate behavior, and she suggested being firm but gentle and respectful—in other words, to negotiate the intimate conflict in a caring and professional way.

Although Jackie's patient did not explicitly use racist terms in his sexualizing of her, he might have thought that as an Asian woman, compared to white women, she was more sexually accessible to him. Controlling images of Asian women include geishas, china dolls, and prostitutes. All these images are hypersexualized, and many include being frail, submissive, and quiet. With these controlling images in mind, I suggest that we analyze Jackie's experience at the intersections of gender, nationality, and race. Although this man was her patient, he was older, white, and male. His assumed access to her was supported by ideologies and material conditions that suggest that older white men have more power than, and entitlement to, younger Asian women. Without institutional support, institutional language to describe this experience, or the time to analyze it, however, Jackie dismissed it by saying her patient must have been "confused."

Nurses labeled patients as confused to explain and justify their sexualized interactions. I observed a variety of situations after which nurses called patients confused. These included times when patients were heavily medicated, disoriented, unfamiliar with their surroundings, unable to clearly communicate, or expressing unexpected emotions like anger or love toward nurses. Early in the study, when I asked about the label *confused*, Bill told me:

> There are different levels of confusion. It's not always from mental disorders. A confused patient can still know who they are and recognize family members, but they may not know what day it is. And it may be an orientation thing, where they just need to be told the date. This can happen to you and me also, if you wake up one morning and are not sure of the day. It might just be that they've lost some time and

space in the hospital, in intensive care. They've been medicated with pain medicine. They've been out for four hours at a time. So there's some confusion there. Then you get to the confusion where the patient knows his name but they don't know anything else. They don't know who they used to be, what they used to do, who their family members are. They don't recognize anything.

The identifier *confused* referred to multiple situations. Patients could be confused for days or could reorient after minutes. Confused behaviors were inconsistent. Patients could be aware of their interactions, bodies, and emotions while being unsure of the date and time. Patients could know names but have no control over their movements.

Indeed, much confused behavior is unintentional, but some patients purposefully act confused. Bill described, "You can tell unintentional confusion over intentional confusion by experience. Experience will yield the answer to that a lot of times. Usually you can smell intent, you know, to harm." Even confused patients deliberately behaved sexually. Over time and through experience, nurses learned to distinguish legitimately confused behavior from purposefully disruptive and inappropriate behavior. Experienced nurses assessed the intent of their patients and adjusted their intimate caring strategies accordingly.

Older and experienced nurses see how sexualized idealizations of nursing persist alongside actual representations of nursing and how these images affect patients' perceptions and interactions. When I asked about sexual interactions at work, Mary commented, "You talk about sexuality! Think about how nurses have been portrayed in the media for so long. Even in movies, how nurses dress up sexy. That's the image. The reality is different!" Patsy agreed that although patients interacted with actual nurses who were wearing baggy scrubs, patients imagined sexy nurses. She said, "They look at the nurse as the nurse with the chest coming out of the uniform, with the tight uniform. I think there is an underlying feeling whenever they look at the nurse. And I don't know—I want to—well, it's nice for younger people to think that way." Patsy expressed discomfort with being sexualized but quickly isolated these interactions as happening to younger people. As a woman in her sixties, she removed herself from the possibility of having to confront sexual interactions involving patients and family members.Older nurses attributed not experiencing sexual harassment to their age. Jody, a nurse in her fifties, told me she did not experience sexual harassment at work because she was older. She said, "Yeah. I don't have that problem. Probably because I'm older and don't have the sweet little innocent looks that these young girls do. I don't know if they have any problems or not, but I don't." Mary agreed and said, "It probably happens with young nurses. It probably happens. See, I'm an old nurse now. [*Laughs.*]" Although some nurses insisted they were too old, other older nurses also told me that patients regularly interacted sexually with them. Even Patsy, who claimed she was too old to be sexualized, discussed how patients sexually interacted with her. She said, "Innuendos, innuendos, sexual innuendos. Patients say, 'Just get into bed with me.'"

Rather than seeing these incidents as inappropriate behavior, many older and experienced nurses described sexualized interactions from patients as harmless flirtation. Mia described a situation with a male patient thirty years her junior. He flirted with her, asked her out, and "made a pass" at her. She gently laughed at him, poked fun, and told him that she could easily be his mother. She was not at all threatened. Angie also described many experiences of patients hitting on her. She described times when patients asked if she was married. She said that in those situations, she did not know what to say, so she always said yes. Patients persisted, asking if she was happily married and if they could go out after getting "out of here." "It is inappropriate," she told me, but "you just blow it off." She described another situation:

> I had one guy who I knew was crazy. He didn't want anyone else to take care of him. He came to the hallway, and I said, "Where are you going?" He said, "I'm looking for my nurse!" So I come, and I say, "You want to see me?" He says, "I want to tell you something." I said, "Okay. What do you want to tell me?" He said, "I really, really love you." [*She laughs.*] I said, "I know, but I want you to get better so you can go home." Then he said, "Yeah, but I want to take you home with me." I said, "No, you can't take me home with you. You have your wife at home." "I don't want her!" It was funny. I got along with him pretty well.

This patient did not bother Angie because she knew how to expertly negotiate his advances. Moreover, she focused the conversation on his care. Angie was accustomed to patients developing feelings for her and was not surprised when it occurred. She skillfully acknowledged this patient's needs in a way that did not disrupt her process of caring for him.

In contrast, Anna, a new and younger nurse, expressed significant discomfort when a patient remarked on her appearance. She said:

> Just last week, a patient in a car accident told me, "Oh, you're very beautiful." I'm like, okay. I don't take that personally. Then he goes,

"So are you taken?" I'm like, "Yes, I have a boyfriend." He goes, "Well, let me know when you dump your boyfriend. I would like to get to know you better." That's not appropriate. And then the other nurses told me, "Oh, you know, that patient said that you're beautiful." I acted like it was no big deal, but I'd just try to stay away from that room. I mean, I'd go in there to make sure he was okay, but other than that, I wouldn't stay very long.

Anna felt uncomfortable with the attention from her patient. She did not expect his affections and did not know how to address the situation. Moreover, Anna did not know how to talk about these concerns with other nurses who told her that she should learn to remain unaffected and act professionally. She tried to act unconcerned, but she still felt discomfort. Instead, she did what many young and new nurses did: she avoided the room and the patient.

Less experienced (and often younger) nurses had trouble determining the intentions of patients. Alicia did not know if her patient, who had "grabbed my breast," knew what he was doing because he "could not follow simple commands." She did notice, however, that "his friend saw him doing it," which made her feel "uncomfortable." Similarly, Nadine described a head trauma patient who explicitly requested her presence while he masturbated in his bed. She explained:

I had a patient who he had a gunshot wound to the head. He wasn't completely present. He was masturbating. And we had this communication thing where one finger was "stay" and two fingers were "go." And he would try to get me to stay so that he could look at me. I told him, "I know you want me to stay." I said, "No, I'm leaving. You can figure this out on your own." It was totally inappropriate. He wasn't all there, but it was hard to deal with.

Just because a patient was confused or disoriented did not mean that nurses felt reassured or comfortable with inappropriate sexual comments or behaviors. They still either had to ignore the behavior or, as in this case, confront it. Nurses had to negotiate intimate conflict, like anger, with patients, and this work was not institutionally recognized or supported.

Patients also made special requests to be washed in their genital areas, not because they needed to be cleaned there, but because they sought sexual attention. Patsy explained how she knew this distinction. She said, "So he kept his gown up, you know. And he wanted you to wash that area, particularly. I knew he knew what he was doing. At first it wasn't blatant; later on it was like his door was open, and he was unclothed." Patsy explained how she determined her patient's motives by assessing his actions over time. At first she was unclear that her patient was inappropriate, but later his persistence became overt.

Experienced nurses refused inappropriate requests for washing. Mia told me, "Sometimes they ask you to wash them down there and stuff, and I just say no, I am not going to do that." Mia has learned over time that there is a difference between caring for the patient and feeling taken advantage of by the patient. In contrast, Carey, a new nurse, described a patient who specifically requested that *she* give him a shower. When she tried to defer to the patient care technician, he insisted that he wanted *her*. She acquiesced, and afterwards he sexually propositioned her. She explained:

> This one guy wanted a shower, and his nurse told him he had to have a shower. But then he wanted me to come wash his back, and the tech was there so I said the tech can do it, and he said, "No, I want you do it." And I was standing right there, and I quickly turned around and did it quick and said, "Now I'm done." I said, "I have to go." And then afterwards he said, "I want a wife; I need a wife. I just need someone to take care of me." How gross.

Carey complied because she wanted to meet her patient's needs, but she was disgusted when he reacted to her in a personal, sexualized manner. She did not know how to professionally negotiate this intimate incident.

Sexualized interactions from patients and family members affect professional intimacy in other ways. Josie described her discomfort with patients who sexually propositioned her, but she did not want to hurt her patients' feelings. She said, "It's more uncomfortable with young men that they will just say inappropriate things, or ask you out, or give you their phone number. What do you say to that? You don't want to be mean to them. You know, it's so hard." Josie's discomfort resulted from not knowing how to confront sexual interactions involving patients without harming them. Her unwillingness to embarrass or "be mean" to patients overshadowed her uneasiness.

Sexualized interactions from patients affected nurses and whether or not they could establish intimate trust and maintain professional intimacy. Although some individual nurses told me that sexualized interactions involving patients and family members were infrequent, my study demonstrates how sexual interactions involving both confused and aware patients pervaded hospital nursing. Nurses described experiencing sexually intimate interactions from patients and family members while simultaneously denying that the interactions had occurred. I assert they did this in part because they thought of sexual interaction in terms that kept it private, not social and natural, not socially constructed. In addition, they maintained a false binary to explain the motivations of patients: ill people are dependent and cannot make choices over their lives, whereas independent people have agency. These false splits—sexual intimacy from public work and dependence from agency—masked how experienced nurses negotiated this specific kind of intimate conflict to regain intimate trust.

Sexual Interactions between Patients and Visitors

In addition to navigating sexual interactions involving patients, nurses witnessed patients sexually interacting with visitors. Depending on the acuteness of their illness, their age, and how permissive their nurses were, patients slept with visitors and engaged in sexual behaviors such as kissing and oral sex. For example, Tammy told me that she "walked in on somebody having a blow job once. It was a family member who had stayed the night." Melinda had "patients and visitors in the shower together." Jill described how she entered a patient's room in response to a medical signal and found herself interrupting an intimate moment: "I was taking care of a guy with a bowel obstruction, and he had a NG tube, and his girlfriend came in, and I left them alone. And the beeper goes off; I walk right in, and the curtain is wide open, and she is sitting there, giving him a blow job! I didn't say anything. I didn't do anything. I just walked out. I let them be together for a bit and forgot about it."

Jill was not bothered by this demonstration of sexual intimacy between her patient and his guest. Because she did not need to administer any medication or procedures in this case, she could turn around, walk out, and "forget about it." Jill avoided conflict and discomfort, but negotiating this kind of sexual intimacy while ensuring quality care was not always this smooth. Nurses had to consider how visitors could disrupt the care process as well as how they might enhance it. In other words, sometimes visitors helped patients feel more comfortable, but sometimes visitors were in the way. Nurses told me that although they had witnessed sexually intimate interactions at all hours, they were infrequent during the day because doctors, physical therapists, lab technicians, social workers, and other hospital staff were constantly moving in and out of patient rooms. Sexual and other physical intimacies happened most often during the night shift between 7:00 p.m. and 7:00 a.m.

Visits from friends and family members were good for the well-being of individual patients but disrupted sleep and medical care and could potentially bother other patients in the unit. Night nurses said that ensuring that patients sleep was their first priority, and as much as they could, they facilitated sleep on the unit. I watched night nurses in all units lower their voices and dim the hall lights after 9:00 p.m. or 10:00 p.m. They knocked on doors softly before entering rooms. They were careful to ensure the comfort of other patients in semiprivate rooms and patients in the unit. Danae said, "You do what is beneficial to the patient. We allow people to stay until 10:00 or 11:00 p.m. If they can be quiet without making noise or getting in conversation, that's fine because the next person has just as much right to their privacy and their rest." Josie agreed, "But most hospitals are semiprivate rooms, and for the sake of the other patient, you know, you just can't let a person of the opposite sex stay." Melinda explained that visitors come to the hospital at, "eleven thirty, twelve o'clock at night and we have other patients in the room sleeping, and we've had six, seven, you know, eight people in a room at a time."

Sometimes, patients planned their intimacy with spouses. For example, I overheard one patient tell a day nurse that her husband would be coming to visit her that evening. Excited, she said, "He wants to sleep in the bed with me." The nurse responded that this was the night nurse's decision and that it might be a "weight issue." I was surprised to learn that the nurse's concern was a "weight issue" (how much the bed could hold) rather than something that addressed the issue of intimacy more directly. When I asked her if it was appropriate for the patient's husband to sleep in the same bed as the patient, she told me the night nurse would make that decision. The day nurse evaded the issue of intimacy because she knew that she would not have to confront it.

Not all night nurses agreed that it was the responsibility of night nurses to determine whether visitors could stay the night. One evening Mia expressed annoyance to me because the day nurse had "allowed" a male patient's girl-friend to sleep with him. I had just observed a woman in a slinky, shiny outfit arrive on the floor at approximately 9:00 p.m. when I followed Mia to her patient's room and saw that the visitor had climbed into bed and snuggled up to the patient. Mia pulled me aside and said, "Here's the deal." Mia explained that she still needed to go into the patient's room with or without the visitor in bed. Mia told me that this behavior was "unacceptable," but she felt pow-erless to confront her patient because he had already received approval from the day nurse. As Mia and I both overheard the patient and his girlfriend gig-gling, I asked her if she felt like she was entering their bedroom. Mia nodded and shrugged at the same time. She said, "Yes, but what can you do? They know this is a hospital. You don't do that. I just have to close my eyes." Mia said it was unacceptable for patients to sleep with visitors. She did not like these kinds of intimate conflicts, but she felt she needed to comply. As in the case of patient slurs and pickup lines, patients demonstrated agency when they were sexually active with their visitors, and to ensure quality care, nurses were in the position of balancing their intimate wants against their intimate needs.

Patient satisfaction did not always translate to quality medical care; that is, the wishes of patients were not necessarily in their best medical interest. Depending on the illness, the injury, or the potential emergency, nurses consistently negotiated the physical closeness between patients and family members. Nurses were concerned not that patients were having sex in their rooms but whether this activity was safe for their patients. They used discretion and thought mostly of their patients' well-being. Tom explained:

> We let them stay. We kind of, you know, turn the other way when visiting hours end. Because that patient has been there, you know, for three weeks, or whatever, you know. Yes, that's also part of health care. And if I can find a room where it's—where it's not going to, you know, um, offend anybody, you know, a roommate next door, or they have their own room of their own, you know, that's okay. You know, we usually allow it. But like I said, it all depends on the patient's health risks. If that's a fractured femur, I cannot risk, you know, having that, you know. It's life versus having a sexual encounter. I mean, what do you choose, you know? I mean, do you want your patient to be alive?

As was the case with Jill, it was not that Tom did not want his patients to be physically and sexually intimate with visitors. It was his job to think about how and when visitors could be present without risking his patient's healing and recovery. Here Tom, like other experienced nurses, did not think it odd that he considered the sexual needs of his patients, he simply incorporated these issues in his planning for the night.

Most nurses agreed that a visitor could sleep with a patient if the patient had a private room and there was no medical threat, but it could be awkward for nurses, especially for those who were inexperienced. Josie described that she hates "feeling mean" when she finds visitors in patients' beds. She did not want to tell them no mostly because it was awkward to discuss the subject.

> And, as much as I don't want them in the same bed, because I need to come in and do my checks, and it's just awkward; it's awkward for me. Like, have to push an IV while one person's arm is around them. [*Laughs.*] But I don't ever tell them to get out, because [*laughs*], again, it's awkward on my hand. I don't want to deal with one extra thing of somebody being upset because they're not sleeping in the same bed.

"And really, when it comes down to it, is it really hurting me? But it's a little uncomfortable, and I don't feel like I can say anything.

Josie felt conflicted between being the professional nurse at work and in charge of patient care and the nurse who did not want to impose on someone else's privacy. Josie expressed discomfort with intimacy between patients and their visitors but tried to rationalize it by suggesting that it did not harm her. At the same time, she was burdened with determining how to balance quality care with patient satisfaction. She felt like she could not say anything because she did not want to offend patients or make them dissatisfied. Her job was to ensure comfort and patient satisfaction, even when it was at her expense. How Josie took time and energy to consider and negotiate intimacy to ensure patient satisfaction is unacknowledged labor.

In contrast to Josie, some nurses avoided negotiation altogether and simply enforced hospital policy. These nurses said that the practice of visitors sleeping with patients was completely "inappropriate" and insisted that family leave at 8:00 p.m. Danae did not allow family or friends to get in bed with patients. She said it was against hospital policy. She told couples that sharing a bed could interfere with emergency care. She told friends and family, "Your loved one is my priority." Similarly, Anna described a patient with a crushed leg who was also experiencing a high temperature that could complicate the injury. One night, Anna found her patient's wife in bed with him. She said, "I remember seeing her in the bed. I said, 'I can't really have you in the bed. I know he's your husband, but he's running a high temp, and your body heat and his body heat make his temp stay up.' And I didn't have a problem." Danae and Anna justified their decisions by educating patients and visitors on medical risks. That nurses needed to justify their decisions demonstrates the pervasiveness of a culture of patient satisfaction. Moreover, these interactions illustrate how nurses must negotiate sexual intimacy, hospital regulations, and quality care of their patients.

Nurses like Jill and Tom knew they had to consider how their patients might be intimate with visitors, but tried to focus their efforts on medical care. Other nurses like Mia and Josie felt discomfort with negotiating patient-visitor intimacy, but deferred to patients because they did not want to initiate a conflict. Still other nurses like Danae and Anna relied on institutional rules to help them navigate the balance between professionalism and intimacy. Eva, one of the more experienced nurses I spoke with, did not strictly enforce institutional rules but also did not avoid patient intimacy. Instead, Eva negotiated with patients and families as a way to balance medical and intimate needs. When I asked Eva if she strictly enforced visiting hours, she said, "Oh no, I slide. Sometimes family members don't get off work [in time], so I'll say, 'The patient is going to need to sleep at 10:00 p.m. Would you mind waiting in the waiting room so she can get some sleep?' Or I'll say, 'Are you aware of the visiting hours?' Sometimes we might say things that are inappropriate, but we have to remember to do customer service."

Eva risked patient satisfaction to ensure quality care, but maintained "customer service" by negotiating the emotional and medical needs of patients. She understood that the schedules of visitors did not necessarily coincide with hospital rules and bargained with patients and visitors to offer patients time with visitors. Eva knew that contact from family members and friends contributed to quality care and also increased patient satisfaction.

One way that Eva negotiated the balancing of quality care with patients' needs was to negotiate patient-visitor intimacy by speaking with visitors in a respectful way. She enlisted visitors as collaborators in the healing process. She did not deny rules or personal intimacies; instead, she asked families to help her. She explained, "It is usually the younger kids and the women who like to be in bed with the male patients. They don't want to be sexual. I [say to patients], 'I understand that she wants you next to her, but [I say to visitors] do you mind sitting in the chair? Because if something happens to him, I'm responsible.' I ask these women, 'Would you consider that for me?'"

Another strategy to balance intimate care with patient satisfaction was to explain the meaning behind the policy: "All the time, I have to explain to them the policy that they can't stay because this patient has a roommate. 'It's like your bedroom,' I tell them. 'Would you like a strange person to be in your bedroom? It is nothing against you, but my job is to make everyone safe and to keep these patients safe.'"

In both examples, Eva educated patients and visitors on her care process. Typically when nurses talked to me about how they learned to educate patients, they referred to educating patients and family members about illness and aftercare. When Eva asked visitors to help her, she explained what she needed from them in order for quality care to occur. Eva strategically involved visitors in her care plan and chose to involve them in a way that helped her best meet the patient's needs. She balanced professionalism and intimacy to help give patients and visitors agency, but at the same time maintained authority over care.

All this said, even when nurses did their best to negotiate intimacy between patients and visitors, patients did not necessarily listen. Eva explained how patients continued to be sexual after she left the room. She told me that she became frustrated knowing that there was little she could do to change the situation: "I can't do anything; whatever the patient says is right for the patient. You just have to—you can't be anyone's mother. You try to give them an example, but it doesn't work. And it's hard, it's hard, and then you have to bring in the forces—the supervisor, your team leader: 'Can you go talk to this patient?' You are trying to take care of the patient. Nurses don't have time to negotiate things like that." Here is another conundrum that nurses face when providing professionally intimate care. If it is not recognized or shared labor, it can be extremely burdensome for the nurse.

Conclusion

Patients and family members exhibited entitlement to their nurses in part from familiarity with their nurses and in part from a hospital culture that emphasized patient satisfaction. In times of intimate conflict, patients expressed harmful and harassing behaviors, which nurses managed as a part of providing professionally intimate care. Intimate conflict, I found, emerged as a part of professional intimacy and challenged common understandings of professional labor and of what it means to be caring. Providing intimate care was not always inherently good or safe for nurses. This second stage of professional intimacy, intimate conflict, challenged any notion of care as moral action because resolving conflict required more than making ethical choices. Nurses needed to be prepared, skillful, and strategic while providing intimate care to patients. Professional intimacy required that patients express themselves, because nurses need patients to trust them in order to provide the best care. In addition to expressing ordinary medical, care, and service needs, patients expressed entitlement, anger, and sexual desire, which were produced in part by familiarity gained from intimate trust and the hospital's focus on patient satisfaction. To provide quality care, nurses both encouraged professional intimacy and professionally responded to patients' intimate needs as defined by patients and family members. Even when they felt discomfort, nurses found time to facilitate an environment that was safe and comfortable for patients. Although nurses were at best uncomfortable and at worst harmed by these interactions, nurses managed their own physical and emotional discomfort in their professionally intimate care of patients and family members.

The intersectional approach continues to be useful for finding patterns that shape exploitative work experiences for women of color and contribute to social and economic meanings of commercialized intimacy. Women of color nurses had to navigate controlling images at the intersection of race and gender during intimate conflict as they did during intimate trust. Mary stifled her disgust at how her patient explicitly compared her to his mammy whom he had as a young boy. In this case, Mary's patient established intimate trust with her while she was "cleaning him up," but Mary had to work through her feelings of conflict in order to maintain this trust. This is the intimate conflict for Mary. She had to reject herself to do her job. She is not only performing emotional labor and body labor; she is performing "mammy." This interaction is not harmful only to Mary; it has social and economic implications constructed at the intersection of race and gender. First, like other women of color in my study, Mary's patient dismissed Mary as a nurse. Instead, he symbolically demoted her to mammy, a controlling image that reinforced the idea that women of color are naturally subordinate to white men. Over time, these kinds of perceptions could have serious implications for Mary's job and for the relationship between women of color and professional nursing. Mary used body labor and emotional labor to work through intimate conflict in order to maintain intimate trust with her patient, but this labor was invisible to her patient. Instead, he viewed her as unprofessional and naturally caring, when she was actually extremely professionally intimate. His perception of Mary could contribute to normalizing the exploitation of women of color in nursing because it reinforced controlling images and it failed to recognize Mary's skillful and expert contributions to quality care.

When I use the intersectional approach to analyze Jackie's experience, I reveal another example of how intimate care is constructed at the intersections of race, gender, and nationality when some social identities make meanings of others. Jackie's patient wanted two things: a hospital with only white people and an English-speaking nurse. His construction of intimate trust was through an intersection of race and nationality (white and American) and each identity was interchangeable with the other. White meant American and American meant white. This intersection is common and fuels anti-immigrant sentiments in Arizona and other states, which contribute to Jackie's experiences as an immigrant nurse. It also shows how social identities reinforce each other and are interchangeable when creating exploitative work conditions. As in Alicia's case in Chapter 3, Jackie's patient understood her language abilities by focusing on her accent as a marker of nationality *and* race. As in Mary's case in this chapter, the patient caused unfair and additional labor for Jackie. Jackie had to try to work through this intimate conflict to maintain intimate trust with her patient. Here, intimate conflict is much more than body labor or emotional labor. Jackie had to accept her patient's needs, compartmentalize his racist and xenophobic assertions, and emphasize herself as English-speaking.

Finally, there were many more cases in this chapter that could have suggested an intersectional approach, but my data (observations and interviews) did not give me the material to do this analysis. If I had had more time,

I might have been able to ask additional questions that could have given more insight into these intersections. As it stands now, however, I am left wondering: Were Joyce's and Nadine's experiences of unwanted sexual attention from patients specifically shaped by femininity and whiteness? Was Lori's experience of body labor shaped in part by her identity as Latina, at the intersection of femininity and Mexican American? Did Carey's patient want her specifically because she was a nurse, African American, or at the intersection of race and gender? When Carey told me that her patient came on to her by saying "I just need someone to take care of me," I immediately thought of the mammy controlling image. I rejected this analysis when she told me that he "wanted a wife" because "wife" contradicts the image of "mammy." I share these examples to contribute to the discussion of my process of the intersectional approach, not just my conclusions. Also, I hope that these questions inspire other scholars and activists to consider how similar questions might be posed in their work.

Nurses simultaneously denied and described verbal, physical, and sexual harm from patients in part because they receive little or no educational training on these interactions or how to handle them. In addition, hospital policy and administration responses to these incidents encouraged patients to feel entitled, which led to work arrangements that overburdened nurses, limited how nurses conducted professional intimacy, and saved the hospital money in that it did not have to employ resources to deal with these conflicts. Nonetheless, individual nurses learned how to manage interactions over time. Teams of nurses also collaborated on informal strategies. How nurses managed and negotiated boundaries with patients and family members during intimate conflict is the focus of Chapter 5.

5

Individual and Collective Intimate Strategies

atients and family members engaged in harmful and harassing behaviors, which I term *intimate conflict*. Nurses managed these interactions as a part of professionally intimate labor. Although the hospital administrators in my study appreciated nurses and care as an institutional value, nurses generally handled intimate conflict on their own. They employed individual strategies, such as ignoring the conflict, confronting the conflict, and negotiating interactions with patients and family members. Sometimes, however, they also worked together, collectively strategizing through the support of charge nurses, the practice of switching patients, and the sharing of knowledge with each other.

In this chapter, I explore what I call collective intimacy. Collective intimacy refers to how nurses collaborated to professionally define and enforce boundaries that addressed intimate conflicts that resulted from attaining intimate trust from patients. To emphasize the strengths of collective intimacy, I show examples of individual strategies and collective strategies that nurses employed to encourage and maintain intimate trust with patients and family members.

Institutional Response

Nurses had little institutional support to address intimate conflict. Although institutional policies prohibited patients from sexually and physically harassing nurses, nurses did not access the support of these policies and procedures, because they perceived them as unclear and irrelevant to their work with patients and family members. The primary institutional recourse available to nurses for intimate conflict was the zero tolerance policy against sexual harassment, which prohibited verbal, physical, and sexual harassment by patients. However, in the history of this policy, no complaints against patients had been made. Moreover, nurses did not mention the sexual harassment policy as a viable strategy when dealing with harassing patients. Even when I specifically asked about the policy, nurses dismissed it and talked about something else.

Nurses did not use policy to protect themselves from intimate conflict, because they prioritized individual patient satisfaction over general policies, such as those about visitor hours. For example, nurses referred to visitor hours to establish boundaries with patients and guests; however, nurses did not always follow these guidelines, because each unit enforced policies to meet patients' individual circumstances. Tammy, an experienced night nurse, explained that when she started working at the hospital, she observed how other nurses enforced visitors' hours so that she could learn from them how and when to enforce this policy. She previously worked in a psychiatric unit in a VA hospital and was accustomed to strict enforcement of policy. "I came in at a really funny spot," she said. "You see, a lot of those old nurses are just so passive, and they don't do anything about anything; and so I really didn't know where administration stood with all that. And I wasn't going to be the new person creating trouble. But now that I've been there a while, and now that I've talked to the unit director, I just tell those [visitors] to go home."

New to the unit, Tammy did not automatically follow policy, because her colleagues were lenient, and she did not want to disrupt the collective unit culture, even though it contradicted her individual practice. She talked to her supervisor, not because she did not know how to handle visitors or because she wanted to follow the rules, but because the unit's practice seemed to contradict her own.

Nurses also lacked the time to use formal, institutional measures to address conflict. Josie said that she incorporated intimate conflict as part of her work because she could not take time out of her busy schedule to file a report. "Would I ever report it? No. I just deal with it as part of my day. And I don't have time to report it. You know. [*Laughs.*] I'm just like, ignore it and go on with my day." Like Josie, most other nurses did not think that institutional policies applied to their interactions. Because they felt that policies and procedures took too much time, they paid little attention to policies and found ways to cope with what they considered individualized situations.

Although some nurses preferred to assess the needs of individual patients, their own workload, and the culture of their unit to determine their response to patients, other nurses thought that institutional negligence increased intimate conflict. Brett explained: "But what's really worse is when the organization or the unit does not take any type of action. And they perpetuate that behavior from patients because they always coddle the patient, tending to whatever's upsetting them. And I believe the more we do that—the more that we allow this type of behavior from individuals—the more we need to correct that type of behavior. Not necessarily discipline, but correct it."

Brett held the hospital accountable for emphasizing patient satisfaction to such a degree that nursing work suffered. He did not see intimate conflict as inevitable. He thought a collective, institutionalized response would help correct the problem because it would set a tone that would discourage intimate conflict. Helen agreed that nurses had "no recourse" when they encountered intimate conflict with patients and their family members as part of their work. Moreover, she asserted that failing to correct conflict reinforces negative behavior from patients. She described how her director's focus on the patient allowed the patient to continue treating nurses poorly: "[My director] went in and held [the patient's] hand, day after day after day, which, to me, promoted that [the patient] treat us like shit all the time. So it comes back to that customer service." Both experienced nurses, Helen and Brett argued that if left alone, intimate conflict would worsen and that, rather than handling intimate conflict individually, nurses should be able to access institutional support.

These nurses thought that their administrative leaders, who happened to be women, did not handle intimate conflict well. For example, Helen attributed her director's and other administrator's inability to address conflict to traditional feminine norms: "I don't even feel like my own director can go in and handle it appropriately or satisfactorily because of her personality. I think there's a generation difference. I mean, [sighs] some of them are as old as my grandma. They weren't brought up to be confrontational or strong women. And I think they don't have it in them to do it."

Helen thought that nurse supervisors viewed themselves as passive, and so they did not confront harassing and harming patients. She was not alone. Although providing care often includes managing intimate conflict, acts of caring are generally defined through traditional feminine characteristics such as being soft, compliant, and deferential. It could also be that nurse supervisors did not feel they could confront harassing patients without appearing disrespectful to them. In either case, administrators failed to systematically address patient conflict.

Administrators may have felt pressured to respond to intimate conflict in traditionally feminine ways, or nurses may not have been trained to handle these interactions. In any case, nurses often focused on ensuring patient satisfaction and intimate care themselves. This added to the burden of invisible labor nurses already carried, but it made sense to nurses to negotiate intimate trust and conflict on their own.

Individual Strategies

Many nurses described their work as individualized. Each had his or her own license, patients, and practice. Similarly, nurses described how they negotiated conflict in individualized terms. Experienced nurses seemed to "naturally" know how and when to set boundaries with their patients, and new nurses quickly learned that this work was important. In contrast to ideas that care is a "feeling" or an "intuition" that a nurse hones over time, boundary making is a series of strategic decisions that includes avoidance behaviors, confrontation, and negotiation with patients and families.

Setting Boundaries

Nurses saw "boundaries" as important in their practices but were vague in their definitions of exactly what they meant by "boundaries." They characterized boundaries as personal traits, which confused new nurses, mystified this labor, and did not use institutional resources most effectively. When I asked nurses how they addressed intimate conflict, experienced nurses like Jill quickly said, "You just have to ignore it or tell them that their behavior is inappropriate." Bill, a senior nurse with over ten years of experience, advised, "But you want to use your intuition and smell those things to sniff out the problem." Although she had only two years of experience, Melinda agreed with Bill. She explained how she identified and managed conflict with her patients by using her own judgment:

> I think I'm a pretty good judge of character. I feel that I can sense when someone is joking or someone wishes to pursue it further, or someone might be hateful. Then, depending on where it's coming from, is how I feel if it's appropriate. I could have an old man say, [*imitating old man's voice*] "I'd like to take you home, you know. You could be my wife." Whatever. And then I could have someone else tell me the same thing, and it could be completely inappropriate.

Although these nurses disclosed that they set boundaries with patients and family members, they characterized setting boundaries as a personal attribute, not a skill that nurses developed over time. Even when nurses described their skills in this arena, they attributed it to working with patient populations known for conflict, such as prison inmates or psychiatric patients.[1] For example, Tammy, an experienced nurse, explained why she did not encounter inappropriate behavior. She said, "Probably not so much with me because of all of my psych experience. I have pretty good boundaries." Although it is likely that Tammy's experience with psychiatric patients helped her develop boundary skills, she did not address how she developed these skills and how her experience with all patients informed this process.

Mia explained how she developed boundaries over time and through her experience on her unit. Her description emphasized the intimate nature of boundary making:

> What I do is I still get close to them in a way, but there is a line, and I don't know how I draw that line, not to get so involved. I don't know how to tell you exactly how to separate yourself. I don't try and cry anymore when they're hurting. I used to hold their hands, and when I knew that they were Christian, I would pray with them. I still do. I still do but not to the point that [*pause*] I would go to their house and visit them. [*She laughs, a little embarrassed.*] I used to do that. You have to protect yourself.

Mia discussed the importance of boundaries and explained some strategies such as not crying and not going to former patients' homes. At the same time, she could not pinpoint the exact nature of her boundary making. This could mean that boundary making was unique to her, a natural personality characteristic. Alternatively, her inability to explain how she set boundaries could simply reflect a lack of language for this practice, a language that might be developed through an institutional or collective focus on the how-to of boundary making.

Other nurses emphasized the importance of boundaries to protect themselves from harm. For example, Jody said, "Because I really try to have more of a professional relationship with people. Once they know that you're not professional, they will take advantage of you." Melinda described how she began each shift by presenting herself formally to patients and then over time she was more comfortable exhibiting compassion and sensitivity. Her experience illustrates the professional work of boundary making:

> I think I make it clear that this is my job. I talk about what we call a plan of care. I'm pretty formal when I first introduce myself. As the night goes on, and I get to know my patients, I soften up a little bit; you might see the caring side of me. It's not that I don't care at first;

this is still my job, what I do. I like what I do. I love what I do. I'm
here to give you the best care possible. But [*pause*] that's a boundary
you place there. It's how you present yourself and take care of yourself.

Melinda is a caring nurse, but how she set boundaries challenged the idea
that care is a personality trait. Traditional meanings of care suggest that care
is static and that there is only one way to express care. Moreover, to be caring
is an essence, an intuition, almost accidental. For Melinda, however, care was
purposeful. She decided when and how to show "softer" sides of herself to her
patients. This purpose helped reveal the boundary-making work in care and
helped show how nurses and patients constructed care in social interaction.
She also explicitly connected how she was more formal in the beginning as a
way to ensure that patients would not "take advantage" of her.

Although she did not call it setting boundaries, Andrea also acknowledged
that she showed two sides of herself to her patients: personal and professional.
She told me, "I usually try to talk to them, ease their feelings, talk about my
kids or my husband, but let them know as their nurse I'm professional with
medical knowledge and I'm not here to, you know, shake my behind and
throw them some happy pills." Nurses adopted professional distance to help
them maintain boundaries during conflict and avert potential conflict, but it
could have seemed cold to patients and family members. Nurses knew this;
thus, they balanced formality with a personal, intimate disposition.

New nurses who had not yet encountered intimate conflict from patients
or family members knew that they needed to learn boundaries because other
nurses told them that this was important. Carey told me she would "handle"
a patient if he continued to make lewd remarks to her. She explained, "I
would have definitely set boundaries and said, 'This can't happen again,' and
then if it had persisted, I would have reported it again." Younger and less
experienced nurses knew they should maintain boundaries with patients but
did not know exactly how to do this. Celia, a new nurse with less than a year
experience, asked other nurses in her unit how to do boundary work: "I'm
learning to draw the line. And I remember they were like, 'You need to stand
up for yourself.' I told them, 'I can't.' They said, 'Oh, you'll learn. [*Laughs.*]
It's something that takes time, but you'll learn once you draw boundaries.'"
Experienced nurses talked about the need for boundaries but had difficulty
describing how to do this work and when they learned it. New nurses knew
that boundaries were important but, like Celia, could not imagine how to set
them with patients.

Experienced nurses set boundaries with patients and family members as
a way to prevent intimacy from becoming uncomfortable or harmful. They

balanced their own emotional responses with the needs of their patients. They could not, however, describe how or when they learned to do this. As they did with the meaning of care, experienced nurses took the meaning of setting boundaries for granted. They assumed that each nurse would determine how to set his or her own boundaries through individualized practice. They mystified the collective practice of boundary setting when they emphasized personality traits or individual experience. In contrast, I observed nurses practicing three distinct collective strategies to manage conflict: avoidance, confrontation, and negotiation.

Avoiding Intimate Conflict

Nurses avoided intimate conflict because they wanted to help patients heal and because they wanted to avoid embarrassment to both the patients and themselves. When they ignored intimate conflict, nurses employed a useful strategy to do so. At the same time, when nurses ignored conflict they told me they felt distanced from their patients, which could hinder professional intimacy. I watched nurses who, in order to regain professional intimacy, took responsibility for their patients' bad behaviors, which increased their emotional labor and, sometimes, wore down their confidence. Alternatively, nurses avoided emotional connection with their patients, which minimized the potential for trust building. While ignoring conflict seemed to work for nurses in the immediate situation, it also exacerbated the idea that intimate conflict was an individualized situation, rather than a systemic problem.

Some nurses avoided intimate conflict with patients by accepting responsibility for patients' negative emotions. Jane described how she chose to account for the emotions of her patients to help give them a sense of control in their care. After a patient complained about her, Jane told her charge nurse that she would apologize to the patient rather than switch patients with another nurse: "Well, you know, I'll just go back there, and maybe if I apologize and if I tell them that, you know, I was wrong and they were right, maybe they will feel a little bit better. They won't mind that I'm taking care of them. You know, it might make things better." Jane apologized to her patient not because she felt she provided bad care but to ease her patient's discomfort. Melinda agreed with Jane that apologizing helps avert conflict: "You have to start by apologizing for whatever has happened before. 'I wasn't here. I don't know what happened. This is what I can do for you now.' Never tell them no. [*Laughs.*] Reword it."

Nurses who apologized to their patients might have avoided immediate conflict, but over time consistently apologizing could seem disingenuous to patients and family members. It could also mask potential harmful behaviors from patients to nurses. Moreover, it could backfire and make the nurse seem less professional and less skilled to the patient and family. This last consequence could affect women nurses differently. I observed nurses employ this strategy across racial and nationality differences; however, I cannot help but speculate that the consequences for women of color nurses would be worse than those for white nurses. Women of color nurses already risked being seen as unskilled and had to prove that they were nurses, whereas white women nurses carry that identity in their invisible knapsack. For white women nurses, it was never questioned that they were nurses. They do not have as much to lose if they apologize for their patient's bad behavior. On the one hand, this practice seems generous and could help facilitate patient trust and quality care. On the other hand, especially if systematically implemented as a collective strategy, this practice would unfairly benefit white nurses compared to women of color nurses.

Many nurses handled sexual interactions between patients and their visitors or sexual statements or actions from patients (directed toward nurses) by ignoring them. If Jill saw that a patient and a visitor were being intimate, she quickly left, hoping they had not noticed her. If they were not being intimate, she worked around the guest: "If there is somebody in bed with the patient, I'll still take care of the patient, come in and out and talk to them. All the time knowing that the other person is not really sleeping in the bed with them; I don't care." Tammy also worked around guests who slept with patients: "I just made a bunch of noise, so they knew that I was in that room. So I just didn't acknowledge it, and any time I went back in that room, I just made a whole bunch of noise. That happens a lot, actually." Josie also avoided conflict by allowing guests to sleep with patients, but unlike Jill and Tammy, she was nervous about encountering intimacy and the potential conflict that could result. She explained, "I guess it would come down to them saying, 'Well, why not?' And I don't have a good answer for that. You know? I really don't. Why not? 'Oh, well, because it makes me feel awkward. So can you not [sleep together]?' That's my only answer, really. I can still give them good care with a patient with someone in the bed with them." Avoiding the issue altogether helped Josie provide care, avoid embarrassment, and avert conflict. It lessened the likelihood for Josie to establish professional intimacy. It also masked the prevalence of this kind of intimate conflict and hid how experienced nurses handled it.

In addition to patient-visitor intimacy, nurses strategically ignored sexual comments from patients to avoid conflict. Chrissy, an experienced nurse, explained why she ignored what she considered inappropriate comments from patients: "I think it is better to pretend. You can tell them, 'I don't like the way you act or what you said.' But then they can deny it and then complain about you." Knowing that her patients could complain about her if she responded to intimate conflict, Chrissy disregarded her patients' actions altogether. Similarly, Bill avoided direct confrontation because he did not want to intensify the discontent his patient was experiencing. "If I just overheard them, I would never bring that up and say, 'I heard you say I was cute when I walked out of the room.' No, now that's just getting stuff stirred up, and I would not want to stir it up." These nurses ignored disruptive patients as a way to prevent potential intimate conflict, but they consequently interacted less with their patients.

Ray, a nurse with five years of experience, described how he decreased the attention he gave to patients over the time of his practice. This strategy helped Ray avoid intimate conflict, but he felt it ultimately affected how patients trusted him and the care they received. At first, Ray spent extra time with patients, relating to them on a personal level, to encourage them to work through their pain and fear about illness or a necessary medical procedure. Over time, his attention waned: "I'll tell you this much. My first two years out of school, I would try to talk to them, get down on their level, really talk to them. 'If you were my dad, this is what I would want you to do.' Somewhere between the third year and now, I don't really argue with them. I'll go to a point, not as much as I used to. I'll just tell the doctor."

Eventually, Ray's initial compassion changed to avoidance. He could not justify "arguing," because he felt it made no impact on their care and only increased conflict, but to avoid this conflict, he spent less time with patients. In addition to spending less time with patients, Ray discussed how his demeanor with patients changed:

> In the beginning, I was real calm, I would try to talk them out of [leaving against medical advice], even if the patient wanted to leave, and I would go through "why you need to stay." Now, I would say I got somewhere [with them] 90 percent of the time. But if it happened now, I'll get you the paper. I get tired of arguing with them. It just got to the point where my attitude was "You are a grown man or woman; it is up to you. Think about it." And then I'll go do something else. I don't try to sit there and coax them into it.

Although Ray acknowledged that his efforts were successful (i.e., he "got somewhere [with them] 90 percent of the time"), he stopped trying because arguing with patients on a daily basis felt unproductive. At first Ray took responsibility for encouraging patients through fear and pain, but then he shifted this responsibility to patients. He respected his patients' right to make choices about their care but cared less about how they made these decisions. He distanced himself from patients to avoid conflict with them, but failing to encourage patients through decision-making processes could have negatively affected their trust in him.

Confronting Intimate Conflict

Experienced nurses individually confronted intimate conflict. New nurses, however, unaccustomed to intimate conflict, expressed discomfort when they responded spontaneously out of anger or frustration. New nurses told me that they felt pressure to handle difficult patients on their own, but did not always know how and sometimes minimized their harm in hopes that patients would focus on their skill. Other nurses called security, but also found this approach ineffective. Finally, although confrontation often worked in the short term, some patients' behaviors persisted so that nurses had to repeat and adjust their confrontational strategies.

Nurses responded to conflict individually because, although they relied on other staff, they thought of nursing as an individualized profession. Nurses were not trained to address intimate conflict as part of their care, but it occurred as part of professional intimacy so they incorporated strategies that varied according to their level of experience. When I asked Mia, a nurse with over fifteen years of experience, if it was fair to assume that nurses addressed patient and family conflict without hospital support, she said, "Yes. Because we just take care of it, and that is the end of it; it doesn't get big, out of hand." She added, "If that person is really bad and harassing and stuff, we get security." I asked her if they ever had to call security. She admitted, "Not really. I have not seen it happen, because we take care of the situation." According to Mia, it would make the circumstances "out of hand" or worse if nurses had to rely on institutional support. She worried that if nurses incorporated institutional support, it would only complicate a difficult situation. Instead, Mia was confident that nurses could and should handle intimate conflict on their own.

My conversations with new nurses confirmed Mia's statements. A new nurse, Celia, explained how new nurses feel this pressure to "handle" conflict: "Because I know I'm new, [that] I'm being judged. That's just any time you're new. I don't think they're intentionally judging me, but everybody always judges a new person to see what she can handle. Am I going to be known as a good nurse or as the one who always needs to be checked because I'm screwing things up? Can I not handle it? I don't want to be the whiney nurse always complaining."

Celia worried that her colleagues would not perceive her as a team player if she complained about patients. Here, she conflated "complaining" with asking questions. She was afraid that if she asked questions, her colleagues would think she was not doing her job. New nurses were caught in a "double bind."[2] On the one hand, colleagues and administrators expected new nurses to learn how to do care on the job because the administrators insisted that care could not be taught in nursing school. On the other hand, if new nurses asked questions, their colleagues became frustrated. Experienced nurses did not have the time or energy to teach new nurses while working an often understaffed shift. Still, both sets of circumstances set up new nurses to fail. They could not learn how to care, and they were unprofessional when they asked how to do it.

To prove her nursing skill, Anna, another new nurse, minimized the harm she felt from patients' inappropriate sexual attention. Although she told me she thought that patients who commented on her appearance were sexually harassing her, she chose to address it herself. "Definitely. Definitely I do. I mean, if they kept going on, then I would ask to be changed. You know, I would take care of it. I mean, I wouldn't make a big deal." What was most important to Anna was to negate her experience of the interaction. Like Celia, she wanted attention to her labor to be about how she handled conflict herself, but in doing so, she risked seeing her situation as unique rather than systemic and pervasive.

Some newer nurses depended on security guards to handle intimate conflict with their patients, even though Mia and other experienced nurses said this rarely happened. For example, Melinda told me that although she knew her allowing family members to stay beyond visitor hours helped her patient trust her and be comfortable, sometimes she faced the delicate balance of keeping her patient happy and keeping her patient physically safe. If family members refused to leave because they felt entitled to be with the patient, she called security.

> I believe in nipping it in the bud before it gets to something that's out of control and we have to call security. You ask them nicely the first time. You let them know what the rules are. And my personal opinion is I don't even deal with it; I just call security. You know, in that type of situation. That's not our responsibility. Our responsibility is that patient and keeping that patient safe. Eight people in a room are not safe. I mean, at eleven thirty at night, twelve o'clock at night. I'm not going, you know, I'm not going to play games.

Melinda used security to confront patients and family members, but most experienced nurses tried to reserve security for dire situations. Elizabeth explained: "If it got to be really bad, and they just didn't listen to the nurse, we would go get our charge nurse or maybe our director. We'd find somebody. Oh, and I think if it got really, really bad, she'd probably call security. And have them come in and try to just give them a little kind of scare or something, but we never had to take it that far."

Experienced nurses told me that calling security was a last resort because staff members on each unit reserved calling security for the worst, most threatening cases, and these rarely occurred. This made sense to me. I could not imagine that security staff could accommodate the possibility for addressing intimate conflict as often as it could potentially occur at a 250-bed hospital. Then I discovered that even when nurses called security, it did not necessarily solve the problem. Helen found security to be reluctant to confront intimate conflict. When they arrived in the unit, they deferred to nurses, asking for instructions on the appropriate response. Helen explained, "We had a bunch of security issues on our floor. And they said, 'Call security.' And security says, 'Well, yeah, but what do you want us to do? You nurses need to tell us when we get to the floor exactly what you want us to say and do with this patient.' Well, most nurses aren't equipped for that."

Nurses were not equipped in part because they were not trained to address intimate conflict care as part of their care work. Nurses were also not equipped because when conflict did occur, it was understood as a unique experience, separate from professional practice. How care is conceptualized as a personality characteristic, not a social practice, exacerbates the idea that care cannot be taught in nursing school or be collectively strategized.

Most experienced nurses often deliberately confronted inappropriate behavior quickly and abruptly. Helen said that she tells patients who exposed themselves to her to "throw a sheet on and cover up." Brett described a time a male patient tried to solicit sexual activity from him. He told the patient, "That's inappropriate. I'm your nurse. I'm here to take care of you. Comments like that will not be tolerated." In discussing situations in which guests are inappropriately in bed with patients, Nadine told me, "You just tell them to get out of bed. 'I'm sorry, that is not appropriate,' you say." Angie explained her approach when patients were inappropriate:

> I had a patient that absolutely refused to tell his girlfriend to go home, and she was sleeping in the bed with him. But since the curtain was pulled, and the other patient was sleeping, it's easier not to rock the boat. But if you are inappropriate, then I am happy to get you a cot,

you know, or a fold-out bed, you know, chair that you can sleep in next to, but, you know, you just explain to them that's not appropriate.

New nurses did not think they could confront patients and surprised themselves when they lost control and did it anyway. For example, out of sheer frustration from constant questions about her sex life, Anna spontaneously confronted her patient: "At first I ignored it, but as the day progressed, he pulled up his gown and said, 'What do you think about this?' I said, 'Knock it off' and just kind of snapped at him: 'I am not a prostitute; I am a professional. Treat me as such.'" Anna shocked herself when she unexpectedly yelled at her patient. Experienced nurses, however, were not surprised at this response, because they learned that intimate conflict sometimes required confrontation for it to stop. Anna's response suggests that new nurses will confront their patients whether or not they feel prepared to do so. This is perhaps what experienced nurses meant when they said that new nurses will learn how to negotiate their own boundaries as they continue shaping their individual practice. When nurses kept their strategies individualized, they also masked the labor required to accomplish the boundary. If boundary setting is invisible, it is easier to say that it cannot be taught. On the other hand, if nurses mark these strategies as something they do as part of their collective professional practice, boundary setting could be taught in school and then mastered on the floor.

Although direct confrontation seemed like a useful strategy, one that was also suggested by administrators, it did not work over time, because patients refused or persisted with inappropriate behavior. Josie explained, "Even though they do go over that—like, 'If a patient asks you out, then you just say, "I'm your nurse, and that's crossing the boundaries"'—it just doesn't work, though, in the real world. They'll still be persistent." Melinda agreed. She repeatedly told patients, "I'm not talking to you with this disrespect. I will not tolerate you talking to me," and many patients never responded. Nadine insisted that one family leave after visiting hours because they were making too much noise. Although the family wanted this closeness with the patient, they disrupted the rest of the unit. She confronted the situation in multiple ways, none of which worked.

You know if you have a family with a ton of kids, and if you kind of make them feel unwelcome, then they'll leave. So if they are making a ton of noise, I'll go in and say, "I'm going to shut the door here because other people are trying to sleep. I'm going to close the door. If you can be quiet—kind of wrap it up. Visiting hours are technically over." Then you have the ones who won't leave. So you get them a cot. And close the door. [*Her tone is resigned and ironic.*] Some family members are there 24 and 7. Those drive me nuts.

Nadine repeatedly indicated to families when they were inappropriate, but still some families—even well-intentioned families—insisted on staying, especially when they felt entitled and did not understand how their behavior could disrupt quality care.

Although nurses sometimes described confrontation in hindsight, as if these interactions occurred in isolation, my observations demonstrate that confrontation usually included a series of interventions that occurred over an entire shift or for days. Elizabeth described repeated interactions with her patient who first harassed a patient care technician and then proceeded to harass her.

I told him it was inappropriate behavior and that we're doing a job. I said, "We're here to take care of you, but we're not here as any kind of girlfriend relationship, or a sexual relationship. My tech is totally uncomfortable coming in here because you've made a few comments." And he said he didn't do anything, and I told him, "Well, she took it like you did. So you have to remember that we're doing a job here. This is our job to take care of you, but you have to be kind of appropriate with us, too, because it makes all of us feel uncomfortable."

Despite her efforts, Elizabeth's patient continued his behavior throughout the three days that she had him. In addition to making sexual comments, he purposefully and repeatedly exposed his genitals to her. At first Elizabeth tried to instruct him on how to comfortably keep a blanket over himself:

He had a permanent erection, and it was painful for him to have the covers over him, and so he'd throw his covers off and just be lying there naked with his big erection. [*Laughs.*] It was like, "Oh, my God." [*Laughs.*] So, I told him, "You know what; I know it's painful for you, but maybe you could put your knees up and put your sheet over your knees when we walk in the room." And he was okay with me for a while after that, but I heard, trickling down from shift to shift, that he was still doing it. And I think he got a kick out of it, really. He was just showing off his manhood.

When Elizabeth realized that he had not stopped the behavior, she increased her interventions. She warned other nurses about him, knocked on his door, and announced that she was entering the room. Elizabeth told me that he managed to stay covered most of the time, and when he did not, she would remind him of their agreement: "I'd pick the sheet up and put it over him. And I'd say, 'I'm covering you up because it's uncomfortable for me to have everything displayed.' You know [*laughs*], just tried a real nice way. So, I mean, what are you going to do? I'd go in each day, and I'd go in and tell him, 'Good morning, Mr. So and So. Remember our little rule with the sheet.' [*Laughs.*]"

Although this patient's behavior affected the entire unit, no one advised Elizabeth to intervene. Elizabeth told me that she knew what to do because she had sixteen years of experience: "I just knew. No. I don't think anybody ever coaches us on that. I really wasn't willing to deal with him doing that and have everything displayed every time I walked in his room. Because it is an uncomfortable feeling, you know. This isn't a porn house. This is a hospital. [*Laughs.*]"

There is a difference between how nurses addressed intimate conflict and how they talked about how they addressed intimate conflict. Although nurses may have talked about confrontation as if each incident occurred in isolation, they consistently incorporated strategies to deal with intimate conflict throughout their work routines. Although Elizabeth did not explicitly say that she negotiated intimate conflict with her patient, she repeatedly confronted her patient, explained the conflict, acknowledged his pain, and attempted compromise. As he persisted in his sexual behaviors, Elizabeth adjusted her approach and also warned other nurses to do the same. Although nurses said they used confrontation individually, experienced nurses like Elizabeth shared the strategies with the rest of the nursing staff. One-time confrontations usually did not work, but repeatedly negotiating with patients could resolve the conflict and maintain a level of intimate trust. This kind of negotiation took time, however, and nurses did not have extra time to spare.

Negotiating Intimate Conflict

Although it took time, nurses who negotiated with patients and family members simultaneously maintained professional intimacy and control over their care. Nadine explained how she set boundaries with families at night by telling the patient "their" plan for the night. She knew from experience that family members who witnessed these instructions tended to leave and told her when they would be back to visit. By negotiating with the patients, she incorporated families into her plan, which both maintained their trust and gave her control over the care process:

> If patients are here for a major surgery, I usually let the family stay so we can talk about what happens. Usually by that time they'll realize that I have business to do. I'll say, "We have to get you a shower to-night and a shower tomorrow morning." And usually they'll realize—oh, this is pretty hectic. And they'll say, "You know what, we'll come back tomorrow morning." And I'll say, "Oh that would be great. So at 5:30 I'll give him a second shower, and then by this time I'll be done, so you can come visit before he goes up to surgery." And usually I try to make them see that "I want you here to visit. But let me know when you are done; then I'll get started," and then that is usually when visit time is over.

Nadine negotiated visiting hours with this family in part by not talking to them directly so she would not seem like she did not want them there. She hoped they heard her interactions with the patient so she could avoid saying she had work to do and needed them to leave. When she had a chance she was sure to suggest good times to visit. She hoped that the family left knowing that she understood how important they were to the patient. Without explicitly saying so, she conducted her work in a way that would preserve professional intimacy. She maintained intimate trust and control over the care of the patient.

Just as Nadine counted on her families to listen to her, Eva listened to the concerns of her patients and then tried to strategize with them to solve problems:

> Listen. Just listen. I'll just sit down and just be quiet in that moment and just let them get it all out. A lot of times when you do that, you have to find out where they're coming from. And second of all, what's the solution? What can we do? I mean, what do you expect? And then when I find out what they expect and then what can we do, okay, and if they're difficult and don't want to do things, "Okay. Let's do a contract. Do you agree with this?"

Mia also took time to listen to her patients and involved them in their own care. She engaged with their concerns and solved problems coopera-tively. Jason agreed that it was important to give patients choices about their care as a way to avert potential or additional conflict:

I think a lot of it is about making choices, giving [the patients] the power. I think a big problem is when they feel powerless. All this stuff is being done to them. They don't know what's going on; they don't know what to expect. Options and freedom have been taken away. Acknowledge their feelings are valid. I mean, that's pretty much the first step, not talking down to them. That's just about letting them know that what they're feeling is okay. And letting them express those feelings. And working with them on their options.

Jason saw that although they may express anger or other inappropriate behaviors, patients typically created conflict when they felt powerless. As a way to avert potential conflict, Jason simultaneously facilitated patients' expressions of their feelings and gave them power through choice.

Although nurses described setting boundaries as a personal attribute—that is, nurses either "have" boundaries or they do not—boundary making is a series of strategic decisions that include avoiding behaviors, confrontation, and negotiating with patients and families. Nurses set boundaries to aid healing, out of respect for the patient, and to avoid conflict. While individual strategies can work, they do not address the larger picture of intimate conflict, they take too much time, and they minimize conflict labor. Handling conflict individually locates the problem of intimate conflict in individual patients, such as patient attitudes, background, and illness. Defining intimate conflict as an individual problem masks the systemic nature of intimate conflict and how it inevitably occurs with professional intimacy.

Collective Strategies

Just as nurses had strategies to address intimate conflict, so did nurse teams. I define nurse teams, as opposed to nursing staff, as nurses who work together on the same shift in the same unit, regardless of permanent or temporary position. Float nurses who were not assigned to any one unit, traveling nurses, nursing interns and students, and other transient staff frequently staffed units and were part of the team on any particular shift. Nurse teams used informal, collective strategies such as getting support from charge nurses, switching nurses, and learning from experienced nurses to address intimate conflict and regain intimate trust.

Charge Nurses

When nurses could not handle conflict themselves, they approached the charge nurse. Charge nurses were the first-line managers in each unit. They managed staff, performing functions including shift assignment, supervision, and general oversight. Charge nurses helped problem-solve and ensured patient satisfaction. Some charge nurses visited each patient, and others—depending on staff availability—provided direct care. Not all charge nurses availed themselves to staff nurses during intimate conflict, but those who did did so because they felt strongly that nurses should not be abused. Lydia, a charge nurse on nights, explained why she made managing intimate conflict her responsibility: "'Because,' and that's the way I said it to this patient, 'Because my nurses do not have to put up with it.' They should be able to work in an environment where they can be truly free to render care to that patient. And not feel like they're on guard, which can actually undermine the kind of care they're going to give to this patient."

Lydia recognized that intimate conflict, and the distance that nurses created with patients as a result, undermined care. She informally created a culture that did not tolerate abuse from patients. "I don't mince my words. I just tell them, anytime it happens, 'Guess what. This hospital does not have to put up with it.' So, we have a right to a work environment that's free of any kind of harassment like that. So that's the end of that. I don't give them options."

In addition to addressing intimate conflict with individual patients, Lydia handled intimate conflict that happened when guests wanted to stay in patients' rooms. She mentioned the visitors' policy but was more successful when she told families that she was concerned about her patients' safety:

> I tell the couple that if they share a bed, then it could interfere with emergency care later. If you find that your patient is slightly short of breath, then, boom, you need to do everything in your power, right then and now, get him to the ICU, correct diagnostic tests, whatever it is. I just explain it to them, "Your loved one is my priority." After I say that, it usually changes things. If you bring it back to the patient, they change their attitude.

As a charge nurse, especially on nights when no other staff members were present, Lydia possessed authority that helped create a culture that supported nurses and patients and did not tolerate inappropriate behavior from patients.

Hospital administrators might consider formally expanding the charge nurse role so that all charge nurses are trained, supported, and granted authority to manage disruptive patients and family members. This would help distribute the burden of intimate conflict off individual nurses by establishing a culture of intolerance of intimate conflict. However, if administrators chose to increase charge nurse responsibilities, they would need to increase the compensation for charge nurses and undertake a reorganization of administrative labor. In my study, unit directors shared administrative responsibilities with their charge nurses, especially if they did not have full-time administrative support staff. In order for the hospital to provide the charge nurse as a resource for managing and averting conflict on each shift, each director would need full-time administrative support, freeing the charge nurse to handle administrative duties relevant only to that shift, such as scheduling and assessment. Moreover, charge nurses would need institutional support for their efforts. Recognizing that intimate conflict occurs in concert with quality care would help charge nurses and the hospital justify interventions, interventions that would ultimately increase overall patient satisfaction because they would facilitate professional intimacy.

Switching Patients

If they were uncomfortable with or felt harmed by their patient's behavior, nurses—especially new nurses—asked to be reassigned. Charge nurses were not surprised by these requests. They happened often and were usually discussed collaboratively on a shift. Many times, women patients, especially older women patients, refused male nurses outright. Sometimes male nurses sensed that women patients were uncomfortable with them. In these cases charge nurses told me that it was easier to give a patient a woman nurse than to address deeply held beliefs and/or fears. Reassigning patients and nurses was a strategy that nurses used to deal with difficult and awkward situations. Roy explained, "We get little old ladies, and I got to flip up their gown or give them a bath, and it kind of freaks them out. They're a little uncomfortable. I'll go get a female. It's all part of teamwork." Nurses incorporated reassignment into the teamwork of the unit. It met the immediate desires of the patient but required the new nurse to establish intimate trust.

Although this was a useful strategy for nurses, nurses feared that if it was overused, they would appear ineffective over time. Joyce told me that as a patient care technician studying nursing, she went to the charge nurse after a patient made a sexualized comment to her, but now that she was an RN, she would handle the situation differently: "But as an RN, I would just tell him, 'You're not allowed to talk to me like that way at all. And if you keep it up, I'm not going to be able to take care of you. Your choice.' And you just have to cut it off right there. And you have to stand up for yourself in such a way that it's not real confrontational. But that—those boundaries are pretty clearly set, and you can do that."

Like most nurses, Joyce thought that the more experienced she became, the better she would be able to handle difficult situations on her own. Although many experienced nurses confirmed Joyce's theory, this thinking still maintains that nurses should manage intimate conflict individually. It also underemphasized how often conflict actually occurred.

Although Joyce and other nurses thought they would not need to switch patients as they gained more experience, the act of switching patients did not necessarily lessen over time. Although she had been an RN for five years, Josie explained that in the worst cases of inappropriate behavior, she asked for another patient. She felt pressure from other nurses to manage the conflict but identified her discomfort as uneasiness with being "tough":

> There've been times, to the point where I've asked not to have the pa-
> tient back because I felt so uncomfortable. It's just to that point where
> no matter what you've said, or you know, and maybe I'm not as tough
> with them. Because some nurses are like, "Oh, I just put them in their
> place and I tell them, and they don't bother me anymore." Or "I just
> give it right back to them." Or something like that. But I don't; I can't
> do that. And maybe it's the shyness in me or something, I don't know.
> [*Laughs.*] I just get uncomfortable, and I don't want to deal with it.

Despite her experience, Josie expressed doubt about switching patients, because she was concerned that she looked like she could not do her job. In a work culture that equated professionalism with individual problem solving, she did not want to seem weak. In contrast, Jackie, a new nurse, appreciated this strategy. "If I feel like this patient is not treating me like a nurse, it's very easy. Just tell the charge nurse which patient, and they will switch you."

Nurse teams that establish switching patients as a viable practice could inadvertently contribute to the exploitation of nurses of color. This is why it is important to think about this strategy as switching patients, not switching nurses. Recall the section in Chapter 3 where charge nurse Roy talked about the practice of switching nurses. Roy was forthright in his discussion of racist and xenophobic patients. He and other nurses told me that white patients would ask to switch nurses based on minority race or nationality. I observed Roy and other nurses comply with these requests because they wanted to keep patients satisfied and did not want to disturb quality care. They did not tell me how this could contribute to inequalities in nursing.

As long as it would not contribute to systematic exploitation and even though some nurses felt that it could appear as a weakness, asking for another patient could be a useful collective strategy. Instead, nurses internalized conflict as a measure of their individual abilities and saw handling patients by themselves as an indicator of good, qualified nursing. Hospital nurses and administrators might acknowledge that working with intimate conflict is a part of providing quality care, rather than keeping conflict labor covert. This would help nurses and also identify the systemic nature of intimate conflict. Although it was intrinsic to professional intimacy, intimate conflict—especially when it was invisible—also prevented professional intimacy, which stifled optimal care. The persistent practice of switching patients did not indicate less skill or professionalism of individual nurses, but rather pointed to the persistent nature of the problem of intimate conflict. Making the practice of switching patients a viable option could lead to a fair distribution of labor, which could ease individual nurse burnout and increase nurse retention.

Experienced Nurses: Collective Mentorship

In spite of an individualized, "handle it on your own" work culture, many new nurses learned from experienced nurses how to provide intimate care, handle intimate conflict, and set boundaries. For example, Jackie learned from Grace, a more experienced nurse, how to deal with patients who sexually exposed themselves to her:

> So once I told Grace about that, and she said, "Jackie, tell me which patient! I'm going to let him know." So she goes up to the room. The thing is he's not covered. So Grace tells him; [*laughs*] she gave him a speech. And then she said, "Jackie, you're not going to let them control you. You're going to go in there and tell him that is not appropriate." And after that, I tell patients.

Before she worked at the hospital, Jackie did not know that she would encounter patients who sexually interacted with her. Not knowing how to handle these situations, she sought the advice from a good friend with more experience. Grace empowered Jackie and taught her how to confront inappropriate behavior, which was all the encouragement Jackie needed to act on her own behalf.

Melinda also attributed much of her practice to more experienced colleagues. In addition to learning practical tips and medical practices, she learned how to manage intimate interactions from patients and family. She explained how she shares this knowledge with new nurses:

> I have excellent charge nurses and nurses with twenty years of experience, and I'm just like, "Okay. What do I do?" You know, and sometimes you have to take a step back and either ask for advice or just say, "You know what, can you please go in there and deal with

him? Or go in and give him medication? Because he's a jerk, and I just don't like him." And it goes back to having a team that you can count on. I mean, there are other nurses, and I've done the same for them—that they're just like, "This patient and I" or "I'm at my wits end." I respond, "Okay. I'll go give them medication." You know, just work together that way.

Although she did not describe it this way, I characterize how Melinda explained sharing knowledge with her colleagues as collective mentorship. Collective mentorship required that nurses felt comfortable and supported when asking questions and sharing advice.

Although extremely useful, the informal practice of collective mentorship depended on the condition that new nurses felt safe asking questions and experienced nurses felt comfortable giving advice. Jody, a nurse with twenty-five years of experience, did not feel that she could assist other nurses with their nursing practices because she did not want to seem disrespectful to them. Nurses generally felt great pride about their individual nursing practice because it was in part how they defined their professionalism. Nonetheless, Jody reacted harshly about a nurse who seemed too gregarious with a patient, but she felt that she could not express her views to the nurse. "Put it on a leash," she said. "But you can't do that. It wasn't my place. If that's the reflection you want on you, fine. But it's not going to be cast on me." Although she disagreed with the nurse's actions, Jody kept quiet.

In contrast, Patsy, a nurse with thirty years of experience, explained how she warns new nurses how to handle inappropriate behavior from patients.[3] "I tell the younger nurses not to go in there by themselves. Always have somebody with them, to take care, care of the patient. You know, things like that." A practice of collective mentorship would need willing participants. At this hospital there was no systematic way to connect nurses who were willing to ask questions and share knowledge. Nurses found each other by working on the same unit, over time, and by coincidence. Also, like any new professionals, new nurses valued the knowledge of experienced nurses, but did not always know the questions to ask. A hospital-facilitated volunteer mentorship program would capitalize on experiential knowledge without overburdening individual nurses.

Conclusion

I observed nurses create professional boundaries with their patients through and around social and economic constraints. They maneuvered a tight line of seemingly personal exchanges, which were individually and collectively produced. For these nurses, this boundary making was labor that required skill, knowledge, and experience. How nurses made negotiating boundaries in intimate situations seem natural was an indicator of their professionalism, experience, and skill. Defined this way, however, boundary making is limited to only strategies used by individual nurses rather than being a collective strategy used by nursing teams. Because they found institutional measures irrelevant, nurses addressed patient and family conflicts on their own. Nurses responded to intimate conflicts individually in part because nursing is defined as an individual practice, which satisfies individual patients.

As for analyzing intimate trust and conflict, the intersectionality approach revealed relations of power in individual and collective intimate care strategies that may have been previously invisible. When nurse leaders suggested that nurses avoid their patients or assume responsibility for patients' bad behavior to avoid conflict, they may have inadvertently contributed to the exploitation of women of color nurses. An intersectional approach demonstrates how these strategies could harm nurses of color. If white patients already challenge the authority of women of color nurses, avoiding conflict might exacerbate this unfair dynamic. In addition, switching patients is different from switching nurses. The only time I heard of patients wanting to switch their nurses was when they perceived their nurses to be immigrants or women of color. On the other hand, many nurses of all races, nationalities, and experience levels asked to switch patients from time to time. It is important to make this distinction because a strategy of switching nurses could be exploitative if it is based in racism, sexism, and/or xenophobia.

Although ignoring patients could be strategic, nurses' *non*-response to conflict perpetuated the invisibility of professional intimacy, conflict labor, and boundary making. It also stifled professional intimacy because nurses spent less time with patients, and the relationships they developed seemed artificial. Although immediately useful, the benefits of confrontation did not last. Confrontation quickly morphed into negotiation because nurses had to repeat and alter their confrontation strategies in response to their patients' reactions. Nurses who negotiated with patients and family members had the most lasting success, but these measures also took the most time. Formalizing collective strategies such as working with charge nurses, switching nurses, and sharing knowledge would acknowledge the systemic nature of intimate conflict—especially as it relates to maintaining professional intimacy—and would keep the responsibility from remaining on the shoulders of each individual nurse.

Conclusion

*A Call for Collective Nursing Practices and
Continued Research*

Consider the following scenarios.

- You are a patient who has been educated on the relationship between intimacy and quality health care. You know that how you
recover depends in part on how your nurse negotiates intimacy and
professionalism. When you enter a hospital that has a reputation
for caring nurses, you know that reputation exists because nurses
are taught to care well and are not simply caring because they think
it comes naturally to them. You understand that your nurse will be
a good nurse because his or her care work will be supported by the
hospital as labor and not just as an institutional value. You know
that care is not just an idea but also an interaction that nurses will
negotiate with you. You understand that your nurse was not born
to care but was trained how to care for you and that this labor
might not always be pleasant for your nurse. You understand that
you might feel pain and mistrust but that your nurse will help you
work through these feelings so you can get well. In addition to
receiving patient rights literature, you also find literature in your
hospital room on how to treat your nurse. You read about behaviors that are acceptable and behaviors that disrupt the care process.
You know that you will trust your nurse but that trust will come
only with effort from both of you. You know you will pay for your
hospital visit and that your nurse will receive compensation for his

or her labor, but this relationship between money and care does not tarnish the quality health care you will receive.

- As a new nurse, you have studied the relationship between intimacy and professionalism in your job. Ideally, you were recruited to nursing not by signs that said "born to be a nurse" but by signs that emphasized care training and expertise. You look forward to caring for others, and you know that your education will prepare you to handle intimacy in the workplace. You are proud that you feel like a caring person *and* that you have caring expertise. You learned in school that there is not one way to provide care; instead, quality health care shifts according to social constructions of identities such as gender, race, nationality, and sexuality. You know that you will professionally care for your patients, and you feel assured that this work will be supported by a team. You are prepared to handle typical abuses that come from intimate labor and patient familiarity with nurses: sexual harassment, entitlement, and anger. If you cannot handle a situation alone, you feel assured that the next right move is to get help from a colleague. Your administrators and directors understand that providing quality care is collective work and you will be rewarded for asking questions and working as a team player.

- As an experienced nurse, you now realize that you are not alone in how you have honed your caregiving skills over the years. You understand that what may have felt like intuition is actually a complex set of specialized skills. You now recognize what you may have thought of as your own, isolated practice of care as patterns of professional labor shared by your colleagues. You understand the relationship between individual and collective practice and can see how giving care is a social as well as an individual practice. You now have additional language to articulate your caregiving efforts so that these efforts, and the efforts of others, are recognized as professional work. You probably already mentor new nurses informally, but now you might begin to strategize how to connect these efforts to your administration's goals of ensuring quality health care. More likely than not, you believe that care can be taught and institutionally reinforced.

- As a nurse director, you are now empowered to continue to support your nurses in their care work. You know that nurses negotiate intimacy professionally and that race, gender, nationality, and other social constructs influence these negotiations. Although patients do not and should not always be expected to notice nurses' labor, you understand the work it takes for nurses to negotiate trust, mistrust, and conflict with patients. Ideally, you work in a hospital that understands care as both a value and labor. You understand that it is an unfair and unrealistic goal to ask nurses to care equally for each patient. Instead, you want each patient to receive quality health care. You, like the nurse directors in my study, care about your nurses, and you want strategies to help them best care for patients.

Nurses in my study *wanted* to care but did not always have the time, the institutional support, or the knowledge to establish and maintain trust with their patients.[1] This is in large part because the rhetoric of professional work does not include bedside care as a set of labor practices that require skill and expertise. At the same time, patients, nurses, and other medical personnel do not see these acts of negotiating intimacy as labor. Instead, they describe them as personality traits that some nurses have naturally. While I am the first to admit that some nurses may seem naturally caring, my study shows how providing quality intimate care is not a natural, spiritual, or ethical act. It is work that requires analytical intellect, skill, and practice, and it is structured in part through social and economic activities.

Nurses show the value of nursing in hospital medicine by minimizing intimacy and emphasizing professionalism. Some nurses did not identify intimacy in their work because they feared that doing so would negate their experiences of altruistic care, which recognized the genuine feelings of kindness and generosity they have toward patients and their families. Other nurses hesitated to acknowledge intimacy because it contradicted mainstream definitions of professional labor. How nurses, administrators, and patients negate professionalism in care work is directly related to how we continue to insist that care is a natural personality characteristic of women, intimacy is distinct from money, and there is just one way to care. The danger of this rhetoric is clear when we consider how it affects whether nurses get the institutional, social, and economic support to provide quality health care to all patients.

My study shows how care is created in interactions and through multiple intersecting social, political, and economic identities. I use intersectionality theory, theories of commercialized and commodified intimacies, and ethnography to analyze how nurses negotiate intimacy in their professional care labor. Without necessarily seeing their labor, nurses do this work mostly because they need to care for patients as well and as quickly as they can. How the nurses and this study make this work visible leads me to argue that "being caring" is a social event. Intersectionality theory helps me explain how care as a social event is shaped by specific ideologies, practices, values, and beliefs.

Professional intimacy provides a gateway to identify bedside care work in nursing as more than just a natural personality characteristic that some nurses possess. This model could be used to teach nurses how to provide bedside care that is professional and intimate. It also challenges the common perception that first, a successfully caring nurse must possess a *natural* ability to care, and second, patients experience good nursing care the same way. In other words, there exists one universal standard for patient bedside care that good nurses inherently know. Through my sociological and feminist analyses of bedside nurses' acts of and ideas about intimate care, I discovered that intimate care in nursing is by no means a "natural" personality trait of "good nurses." The result of my analyses demonstrates that bedside care in hospital nursing is intimate labor that requires expertise and can be taught to nursing students. This expertise includes negotiating intimacy and conflict, both of which change according to intersections of race, gender, and nationality.

I developed the model of professional intimacy to provide a framework for nurses to advocate for better work conditions. Recognizing professional intimacy as legitimate work will facilitate bedside care and, ultimately, increase quality health care for patients. I also hope this model will help illustrate the potential of intersectionality theory to other researchers. Finally, this model will help labor advocates and researchers explain the function of intimacies in other types of work. Studying the impact of intimacy in care work answers some questions posed in the Introduction to this book. Care is not just an ideal or a personality trait. To be a "caring nurse" is one part of a three-part (medical-technical-care) labor strategy to ensure quality health care for patients. New nurses initially seem less skilled at care because they are not prepared to handle intimacy and conflict in care. Experienced nurses leave bedside care in part because they are "burnt-out" from carrying the load of this individualized, invisible labor.

This book has both practical and theoretical uses. Recognizing professional intimacy has significant theoretical implications for understanding the relationship between commercialized intimacy and the economy and for elaborating how intersectionality theory can be used to study everyday life. In addition, collectively recognizing professional intimacy has practical value, helping nurses better understand the shared conditions of their labor. Attention to issues of professional intimacy in nurse training and in hospitals may also increase patient satisfaction and nurse retention, which might help alleviate the nursing shortage in the United States and other parts of the world.

Contributions to Nursing Practices

This research distinguishes the desire to care from the capacity to do nursing labor. Whether or not it is taught, institutionally supported, or assessed, nurses are expected to ensure quality care through professional intimacy. Not all nurses are prepared to handle intimacy in their profession, but all nurses can learn how to do this work. Naming professional intimacy reveals the skills and specialized knowledge required for care labor. Understanding care labor in these terms encourages institutional and educational supports for these invisible aspects of nursing.

I present this research with hope that nurses might use it to advocate for a reorganization of their work space, labor, accountability, and education in ways that will better accommodate professional intimacy; however, I also realize that this research could be used to the detriment of nurses. As health-care costs increase and the nursing shortage persists, administrators could conceivably use these data to argue for maintaining the status quo by celebrating how nurses balance professional intimacy with medical, administrative, and other care tasks without implementing institutional supports. As noted previously, the hospital CEO said to me in reference to the caring abilities of nurses, "I don't know how they do it. I am just grateful they do!" Even directors interested in supporting professionally intimate labor may inadvertently harm nurses. They could add to nurses' already overburdened labor by expecting nurses to formally train each other without compensation or institutional support. They could require additional charts and other documentation to standardize policies and procedures without reorganizing the labor to accommodate these efforts. While taking nurses for granted and exploiting professional intimacy could occur in the short run, it will not help patients or solve nurse burnout or other problems associated with nurse retention. Recognizing professional intimacy could help formalize individual strategies into collective strategies that could be taught in nursing programs and instituted in the workplace.

Instituting a volunteer mentorship program and teaching nurses—at both the associate level and the baccalaureate level—about professional intimacy *before* they reach the bedside would encourage the use of these practices. Other institutional supports could include reorganizing work space, coordinating responsibilities, and dictating, rather than writing, charts. With barely enough time to chart, dispense medications, assess and provide medical care, and give service, nurses have little time to spend with their patients; however, experienced nurses fit professional intimacy into their work schedules. These efforts could be better supported if professional intimacy were recognized as labor and if a majority of their time was not spent being interrupted, charting, and following up on the work of other staff. Documentation and phone calls take significant time and pull nurses away from their patients. Moreover, both nurses and patients want patients to access nurses when they need them, as characterized by a nurses' station that is in the center of the unit, open, where people freely walk and talk. The problem is that nurse accessibility is not the only purpose of the nurses' station, as other staff members—including physicians, respiratory and physical therapists, and social workers—also use this space to conduct their business.

Hospitals could better structure nurses' time by reorganizing space and responsibilities to accommodate professional intimacy. A work area could be created that would give nurses space and time to chart. This would reserve the nurses' station for interactions between patients and family members, which would encourage professional intimacy. Increasing the responsibilities of administrative support staff to include follow-up with staff could also free nurses to conduct professional intimacy. Dictation of charting would save nurses time that could be spent with patients. Finally, hospitals could encourage patients to consider their nurses in their interactions with them. Just as they post patients' rights in all units, they could identify patient behaviors that are detrimental to quality health care. As it stands, nurses are the point people for patients and family members. They are the clinical staff members most likely to catch illness or injury when it turns for the worse. Allowing nurses to conduct professionally intimate work will ensure better medical care to patients—care that could ultimately save lives.

Suggestions for Future Research

This theory of professional intimacy demonstrates the significance of both professionalism and intimate labor in nursing practices. Professional intimacy rejects dichotomous framings of care as either altruism or professional skill to show how hospital nurses use both to provide quality care to patients and families. My research reframes the discussion of what it means to be a good nurse by rejecting naturalized definitions of care, femininity, and whiteness. Instead, my analysis reveals the labor that is required to conduct care in a hospital setting. Rather than focus on whether nurses are motivated to care for either altruistic or economic reasons, my research shows that nurses and patients construct what it means to provide care and also that ideas of care are constructed along lines of gender, race, and nationality.

Future research in the area of professional intimacy should continue to use intersectionality theory to further develop the concept of intimacy as it functions through other identity combinations and incorporating identities not found salient here, such as sexuality, ability, and, although addressed cursorily here, age. The concept of professional intimacy could be studied in other nursing contexts and honed in other professional work such as social service, pastoral care, and education. The theoretical development of professional intimacy could also occur through study of the professional nature of intimate labor in areas such as massage therapy, the sex industry, and the beauty/spa industry.

Finally, the concept of professional intimacy should be studied in the international professional care labor market. These studies should focus on the relationships among race, ethnicity, and migration status in nursing and how nurses negotiate cultural stereotyping and economic discrimination in their host and home countries. Studying how these factors condition the experiences and understandings of professional intimacy will bring us closer to increased social and economic values of professional care work as it occurs around the globe. It is my hope that this book lays the groundwork for such future endeavors.

Appendix A

Why I Define My Research as Feminist

I am a feminist, but I do not consider this identity sufficient to define my research as feminist or to label me a feminist researcher.[1] I define my research as feminist not simply because I chose to conduct participatory research that highlights diverse experiences or because I hope that people outside of the academy find my work relevant to their lives. I do so because three historically feminist ideals ground my work: safety, accountability, and empowerment. In my effort to protect the participants, I maintained confidential data while remaining sensitive to the vulnerabilities and fears of all the participants, including my own. My research was accountable, not just because I reported back to participants but also because I chose topics that affect everyday individuals and groups. My research was empowering because it listened to and strategized with nurses. These conversations highlighted the intelligence and strength of hospital nurses and revealed and challenged institutional social inequalities.

I bridged theory and praxis by choosing my location, in part, because hospitals in this rapidly growing region needed research on nursing. I used institutional ethnography that focused my research on the lived experiences of nurses to help nurses positively change their work environment.[2] I used standpoint theory and prioritized the concerns of participants throughout the study. My data collection, analysis, and dissemination included plans that responded to the needs of my participants—as identified by the participants themselves. I constantly considered how meanings of whiteness, masculinity, femininity, skin color, and citizenship affect intimate labor and influenced the research process. Did these choices make this research feminist and me a feminist researcher?

I am not sure. Many scholars before me warn against assumptions of relying on feminist identity and banking on shared motivations between participants and researchers. For example, Judith Stacey reminds us that intimate encounters in ethnography can lead to exploitation.[3] And Kathleen Blee tells us that the "you know what I mean" that sometimes occurs between women can lead to conceptual confusion.[4] Moreover, in Dorothy Smith's own words, standpoint and intersectionality theories are not in and of themselves feminist. Standpoint theories, at times, run counter to mainstream feminist research.[5]

I continue to have three ambitions for this project. First, I hope that I have revealed the value in providing professional intimate care in nursing. Second, I hope to show that intersectionality is necessary for rigorous research on gender.[6] Third, I hope that nurses use this research to garner improvements in their work conditions that will facilitate the labor of professional intimacy. In this section, I explain the methodological and conceptual trajectory that shaped my research. I changed the focus from sexual harassment to intimacy in professional nursing, largely in response to nurses' understandings of their own experiences. I detail issues of entrée, participant protection, and ethics. I discuss my data collection, analysis, and dissemination. I conclude with final thoughts about why I think this project is feminist research.

Pilot Study

My first lesson in conducting research for this project involved checking my feminist biases at the door. The research in this book was inspired by a pilot study I conducted in graduate school. For this pilot, I compared waitresses' and nurses' experiences and definitions of sexual harassment. Based on the research literature and my own thoughts about the function of sexual harassment, I expected nurses and waitresses to have similar descriptions of sexual harassment on the job. Instead, I found that while both groups described what they considered uncomfortable or inappropriate sexual situations as part of their work, waitresses labeled these sexual harassment and nurses did not.[7] While at first I struggled with understanding how nurses were not sexually harassed by patients, I eventually practiced self-reflexivity and listened to nurses' meanings of nonsexual harassment. I listened, even when their statements seemed antithetical to my feminist ideas. I considered other explanations for sexualized behaviors from patients, and this direction in analysis was fruitful. I found that this difference results from work norms about intimacy, perceptions of clients' intentions, and levels of power in the workplace.[8]

I conducted twenty-one in-depth interviews for this study. In 1994 I interviewed ten waitresses who were diverse by race, sexual orientation, and age. I purposively sampled waitresses from three types of restaurants—with differing price of meals, atmosphere, and clientele—to ensure variance in workplace culture. In 2003, in partnership with 1199P/SEIU, Pennsylvania's chapter of Service Employees International Union, I interviewed eleven nurses diverse by gender, age, and work area at one large urban hospital in Pittsburgh, Pennsylvania. Eight nurses were female, and three were male. All were white, U.S. born, and heterosexual. They worked in different areas of the hospital: emergency room, operating room, intensive care, and obstetrics and gynecology. Their ages ranged from twenty-one to fifty-two.

For waitresses, I asked mostly open-ended questions about work culture, interactions, and meanings of sexual harassment and inappropriateness. I also asked some categorical questions in conjunction with a list of behaviors I defined as sexual harassment—that is, touching, crude remarks, and the like. If an informant responded yes to any of these behaviors, I later asked if she or he would define the behaviors as sexual harassment.

When I began interviewing nurses, I constructed an interview guide that relied on open-ended questions. Since I sought nurses' understandings of sexual harassment, I did not want to impose prescribed categories in the interview. I found, however, that when I did not include some of the prescribed categories that I used with waitresses, many research participants were vague and did not address sexual harassment at all. In an attempt to garner more specific data and allow a better comparison with waitresses, I then asked nurses about specific behaviors. In later interviews, I noticed that I did not need to rely on this prescribed list if the informant led the interview. I coded discussions of behaviors conventionally thought of as sexual harassment, even if research participants did not define these scenarios as such, including jokes, crude remarks, and requests for sexual favors. I also looked for references to behaviors that are not conventionally defined as sexual harassment but that research participants defined as "inappropriate."

My pilot study suggested that cultural understandings, including those shaped by work norms, are important to understanding sexual harassment.[9] The relationship between meanings and culture brings into question whether traditional avenues for recourse against workplace sexual harassment are appropriate in caring professions. My analysis also pointed to the need to understand how nurses' lives outside of work might affect how nurses distinguish between appropriate intimacy and sexual harassment. This suggested that nurses' cultural belief systems shape understandings of work dynamics. This fit recent scholarship by labor sociologists who found that the private lives of workers affect their work lives.[10] Finally, my pilot study suggested that relying exclusively on interview data, especially data from structured interviews, had limited my analysis. Several nurses offered only vague responses when asked directly about sexual harassment; they were more forthcoming in later interviews with more open-ended questions.

Research Design

Since my pilot study showed that interview data alone were insufficient to explain why nurses responded in particular ways to sexualized interactions, why these responses changed over time, and how different work contexts influenced their responses, for my dissertation I decided to conduct an ethnography, situated in global circumstances.[11] Global ethnography attaches globalization processes to everyday life. It is "grounded globalization," which connects local ethnographic research on hospital nursing, for example, to discourses about the global nursing shortage and commercialized care.

I also draw significantly from standpoint theories, which explain the everyday world by prioritizing subjective worldviews and experiential knowledge. This does not suggest that any knowledge is superior; rather, it is a method of inquiry that focuses on the relations between knowledge and power in three ways.[12] First, standpoint theory emphasizes the role of authoritative documents and texts in constructing and normalizing everyday experiences and meanings.[13] Second, standpoint theory focuses on how social locations vary by material resources and realities that reflect oppression and resistance.[14] Third, standpoint theory points to the need to analyze how multiple subjectivities and experiences create knowledge.[15] I used these features of standpoint theory to analyze experiential knowledge from the standpoint of nurses to reveal the everyday world of interactions between patients and nurses. Incorporating knowledge from a position that is "bottom-up" provided a fuller analysis of intimate and sexualized interactions between nurses and patients than would more conventional "top-down" analytic approaches.

Study Site

In the United States, there has been, and continues to be, significant discrimination against Latinos and Latinas, especially in border states such as Arizona. As I completed the writing of this book, Arizona had passed its anti-immigration Senate Bill 1070, and replicate strategies were quickly picking up speed.

Lawmakers in New York, Washington, Nevada, and Rhode Island were reporting plans to introduce new legislation that would increase border security and/or require anyone to carry citizenship documents on their person. Arizona Senate Bill 1070 requires police to detain anyone they "reasonably" suspect of illegal status; police do not need a warrant to stop or arrest anyone they suspect of "being an illegal alien." This puts Arizona Latinos and Latinas at serious risk for racial profiling. While I conducted my research, I lived in Arizona for nine months. While living there, I frequently observed racial and xenophobic acts in my daily life as well as in my research. As I am a white woman who speaks English as my first language, many people likely perceived me as "safe" to share their racist and xenophobic beliefs with. As a consequence, I often heard anti-immigrant ideas from people expecting me to agree with them. I also observed significant patterns of anti-immigration sentiment in my research. The Latina nurses in my study and other nurses who were perceived to be immigrants because of their accents or skin tone faced unique discrimination at the sites of nationality, gender, and race.

The hospital I studied was in a poor neighborhood, with a significant homeless and drug-using population. One of the few trauma hospitals in the state, it was well known for its excellent nursing care and was a midsize hospital that served community residents. Its patient population was mixed: some were wealthy, some were poor, and some were homeless; some were year-round residents, some visited during the winter months, and some were undocumented families who had traveled from Mexico and other Central and South American countries. Most trauma patients were relatively young. Older patients were battling cancer, heart disease, and other illnesses.

Administrators in my study site struggled with providing enough nursing staff to meet patients' needs. The winter I conducted my study was especially challenging, with the highest-ever recorded admissions to the inpatient surgery department; the number of inpatient surgeries in January and February increased 17 percent from the year before. During the Christmas holidays, the management team suited up and provided bedside care, staff converted office space to bed space, and employees came in to work on their days off. Administration struck a partnership with a registry service so that nurses from this registry would be trained on hospital policies. This was in addition to a float pool of staff nurses originally designed to fill shifts of nurses who called in sick, not to fill permanent positions. In early 2007, the hospital planned to employ immigrant nurses from India to help fill their ranks.

With twenty beds, the oncology unit was the smallest unit in the hospital. There were four to five nurses on staff during the day, each of whom cared for four to five patients, and four nurses on staff during the night. Half the patients were oncology cases and half were medical-surgical cases. Oncology was the least diverse floor. Most nurses on this floor were experienced, white women. I interviewed two men and two people of color from this floor. The progressive coronary care unit (PCCU) was the second-smallest unit, but it had a faster pace than oncology. Patients were older, they needed to be moved more often, and some families dealt with end-of-life issues. There were four to five nurses on shift, many of whom were recent hires. I interviewed three male nurses and three people of color from this floor. With thirty-six beds and seven nurses per shift, the medical-surgical floor was the largest unit of the hospital and turned over more patients than any other floor. This unit had the most racially and ethnically diverse staff; many nurses were trained in other countries. I interviewed two men and seven people of color from this floor. With seven nurses per shift, orthopedics was the second-largest unit; it also moved at a fast pace. Nurses on this floor saw two kinds of patients: trauma patients, who typically were relatively young, and patients with alcohol-related or orthopedic conditions, who were older. I interviewed three men and four people of color from this floor.

I selected these units because each attended to different kinds of illness and because they varied in size but experienced similar nurse-patient ratios, involvements with family members, and lengths of patient stays. They also had similar control over who could come on and off the floor, and all units cared for medical-surgical patients. Early in the study, other units expressed interest and willingness to participate. I considered including units such as the intensive care unit, the emergency department, operating, and labor and delivery, but I discovered that these units had distinct work features and cultures that made them too different from the other units for a fair comparison of meanings of intimacy in care work. For example, the emergency department moved at an urgent pace with an open door, so that nurses watched for unknown or uncontrollable circumstances. As the director of the emergency room explained, "it is a very different place," and it is "part of the culture" there to deal with stress by talking and joking about sexual and intimate matters. She said the line between appropriate and inappropriate behaviors blurred and could bias my findings. Similarly, the intensive care unit worked with acute illnesses but had a very low patient-nurse ratio compared to the other units in the hospital. Patients were not alert, and interactions with family were much more intense.

Gaining Entrée and Developing Rapport

As someone new to studying nursing, I consulted many nurse researchers and practitioners while conceptualizing, designing, revising, and implementing this study. I conducted formal meetings (both in person and by phone), had informal conversations, and attended meetings at twenty hospitals and organizations in six states, representing the East Coast, the West Coast, the mountain states, and the Southwest of the United States.

In June 2005, I contacted a state association of health care and a hospital association for a state in the Southwest. They immediately referred me to several hospitals in one of their largest metropolitan areas that they felt would benefit from nursing research. I called all of these hospitals and scheduled visits with two in August 2005. The first hospital was a large urban center with 650 beds. The director of nursing expressed interest in my project. She invited me to the site, gave me a tour, and introduced me to the human resources director. However, my study, particularly its emphasis on sexual harassment, proved to be too risky for the organization. The director of human resources rejected the study, saying, "Now is not a good time."

The director of professional practice at the second hospital scheduled me first with several clinical directors who expressed interest in the project. Many staff nurses were not trained to understand the importance of qualitative research. This was one of the reasons the director of professional practice and other administrators were interested in my study. They hoped to expose staff nurses to the qualitative study of nursing. This first meeting gave me an opportunity to explain my intention to be as little work for them as possible. I took time and great care to express how I would defer to them and their staff to be sure that I would not disrupt patient care or the flow of work. I also met with the vice president of clinical care to share the project goals, methods, and my plans on how to approach ethical concerns. I left my August meetings with an informal approval from the director of professional practice. She gave me an application to complete to secure formal approval. In September 2005, I received a letter stating formal approval and commitment to work with me and also gained approval from the University of Pittsburgh Institutional Review Board.

Although the nurse directors were interested in the project, they had two significant concerns, both of which surprised me. First, they warned me against using the word "sexual" in my project description. They were worried that staff nurses would not listen to me or take me seriously. In this case, I listened to them and replaced the word "sexual" with "intimacy." The nurse directors were right. I had already learned that "sexual" had many meanings for staff nurses in my pilot study. Because I broadened my focus to include intimacy, I also broadened my research lens, which helped me understand and explain nurses' work conditions from their perspectives. It also helped me to see different forms of intimacy, both the extreme and the mundane.[16] The nurse directors also suggested that I eliminate my focus on sexual harassment altogether. This I did not do. Although I would not use the word *sexual* in my initial conversations, it was important to keep an open mind about both harmful and helpful intimacies, in spite of pervasive meanings of care as only good. Second, nurses and nurse directors, all of whom were white, thought it a waste of my time to study race in nursing because "most nurses are white anyway." I did not listen to them. Instead, I listened to the scholars who explain the importance of whiteness in research[17] and who note that studies of gender must include intersections of race and other social identities[18] and that race always enters the research process.[19] I imagined the nurses who were not talking to me during my design; these were nurses of color—black, brown, and immigrant. Both these moments—the decision to eliminate the word sexual and the choice to study race—were feminist because they responded to voices heard and those who were potentially unheard. At the same time, they challenged the idea that we should listen to and take all suggestions of research participants. I think doing this could potentially cause the researcher to fall into a trap of "glorifying" local voices as unbiased or uncorrupt.[20]

In late September I moved to begin my research. I held a second meeting with clinical directors in early October. In this meeting I shared my research plan, asked for feedback and questions, determined the order of units I would study, and scheduled individual meetings to discuss particular issues and concerns for each unit. I asked questions about how to introduce the study to staff, the physical space I could access, the documents I could see, and meetings I could attend. The clinical directors expressed two concerns to me. The first was my use of the term *sexual* when I described my project to the nurses. The second was the possibility that I might interrupt patient care. The directors were very protective of their nurses and did not want them to feel uncomfortable with my presence in their unit. I avoided using the word *sexual* in initial descriptions of the study in response to the directors' concerns that workers would not take me seriously. In addition, I brainstormed strategies with directors on ways to keep my observation focused but still as inconspicuous as possible. For instance, during my observations and conversations I learned the power of "knowing nothing" while on the floor. I told nurses I was simply there to follow them. I let patients think that I was a nursing student. I did not correct patients until they asked me to provide care, at which point I explained that I was not a nursing student and that I would need to get their nurse. When I explained my project to staff and patients, I made statements such as "I do not know about nursing" and "I am not a nurse."

After I received permission from the hospital and guidance from the clinical directors, I began observation. Before observing each unit, I attended staff meetings to introduce myself, explain my study, answer questions, and initiate rapport. Following the practice applied in Mary Beth Happ's 1998 study of interactions between nurses and patients in a critical care unit,[21] I encouraged nurses to let me know if there were particular events, days, or patients that they would not want me to observe. Also, like Happ, I posted notices of the study in communication books in each area, in the family waiting rooms, and in staff restrooms.

I increasingly gained entrée with nurses, patient care technicians, and other clinical staff. In addition to the preparation I completed, I explained the study to nurses on an individual basis and continually emphasized that participants would be protected from harm, that participation was voluntary, that I would follow the nurses on their daily rounds and observe their interactions with patients and family members only with their permission, and that I was there only to observe their work, not to evaluate it or answer questions. I also emphasized that I would not disrupt patient care. I told nurses that I would observe their interactions with patients and family members but would not interview patients or family members or access patient records.

Gaining entrée was affected by my status as a researcher who did not need to comply with institutional norms. Although my observation and inconsistent schedule breached the routine and fast pace that organized nursing work, it gave me a chance to identify these norms.[22] For example, I often attended meetings and staff in-services as they happened during my observation because they were opportunities to meet staff and build rapport. I learned from nurses that my "coming and going" and the fact that "folks never know when I am going to slip in and out" were "kind of creepy." Looking like I did nothing during observation was a second breach in a very busy environment. For instance, a unit director said to me that she wished she had my hours, not understanding that hours of work waited for me after I left a four- or five-hour observation "shift." Other nurses joked with me when I stood or sat during my observations. To appear less conspicuous, I moved in and out of chairs, from one side of the station to another, up and down halls, and out of the way of other personnel, and I took notes.

Protection of Participants

I kept the names of participants confidential throughout the study and afterward in my findings, reports, and papers. I did not include patient identifiers in my field notes, interview transcriptions, or analysis. I encouraged nurses to avoid using patient names or other identifiers during in-depth interviews. I did not include names in transcriptions when nurses disclosed this information in interviews. I also consistently reminded nurses that they could ask me to cease observing at any point in the process. I sought to be as unobtrusive as possible to ensure that participants were comfortable with my presence in their workplace. This meant that I was hyperaware of my presence and how I appeared to staff and patients.

A Typical Day

Nurses practice in close quarters. A typical day in a hospital unit was busy; nurses, doctors, social workers, case managers, secretaries, dietary staff, and housekeeping staff shared work space but worked independently. All saw different patients at different times and completed their own documentation. Half of the patient rooms I observed were semiprivate. Work space in the nurses' station was at a premium, shared with doctors, case managers, pharmacists, physical therapists, patient care technicians, and other nurses. Still, nurses interacted intimately and privately with patients and family members in public spaces—in patient rooms, in the halls, and in nurses' stations. Workers moved up and down halls and in and out of patients' rooms easily and quickly. They also moved through the nurses' station quickly, often without saying hello. They stopped in the nurses' station to make phone calls, receive phone calls, and chart. People generally did not talk to each other unless it was specifically about patients' progress. Multiple conversations occurred simultaneously: about individual patients, about discharges, phoning the pharmacy, phoning doctors, paging doctors, paging nurses, handling calls with families, talking to the social workers about aftercare or long-term care, phoning the emergency department for a new admittance, technicians asking nurses to unhook IVs or provide other care, nurses negotiating breaks, prosthetic and other equipment representatives coming in, and family members asking questions.

Clinical staff members discussed patient progress but could not monitor the process of their work. They did not discuss patient care in their meetings, which primarily attended to policy changes and institutional goals. They lost charts, moved charts, took charts, and spent precious time looking for charts. Staff called on the intercom for nurses who were five feet away in the medicine room or just on the other side of the divider in the nurses' station. Nurses discussed their practice in individual terms, but they needed each other and relied on institutional policies for patient care.

Unlike in some hospitals, where groups of staff members wear the same color uniform and all staff members wear visible name tags designed to help patients and family members distinguish among their caregivers, staff in the hospital I studied wore uniforms of their choosing that varied by color and design. They wore name tags, but often these were partially hidden or turned around, which made them difficult to read. Allowing staff to wear uniforms of their choice inadvertently equalized workers and made physicians, nurses, housekeepers, and patient care technicians indistinguishable from one another. This enabled patients and family members to use gender, race, and nationality stereotypes when they assigned various levels of authority to hospital staff.

Data Collection and Analysis

From October 2005 to May 2006, I immersed myself in the culture of the hospital. I observed, conversed with, and informally assisted nurses and other clinical staff during the day and night hours (800) on four units: oncology, progressive coronary care unit (PCCU), medical-surgical, and orthopedics. I interviewed forty-five nurses: ten (22 percent) were male, sixteen (36 percent) were people of color, and ten (22 percent) were from other countries. I also interviewed ten administrators and educators. I followed nurses and moved away. I listened and refrained from listening. I talked and kept silent. I felt and stayed unfeeling. How did I keep my research flexible yet precise? I tried to practice what Howard Becker calls "following your nose,"[23] but at the same time, I analyzed data that made no sense to my nose, or to my brain, for that matter. I practiced formal and informal reflexivity to monitor these decisions and track emotions not just to tell a story but to be accountable to my own biases.[24]

On both day and night shifts, I observed nurses in the nurses' station, joined in conversations in the staff room, and walked the halls. I attended staff meetings and received policy updates, unit-specific correspondence, and hospital-wide e-mails. When able to do so without disrupting their work, I informally talked with nurses and followed them on their rounds, observing their interactions with coworkers, patients, and patients' family members. I followed nurses on their rounds for approximately 75 percent of my observations. Within one month, I learned it was most useful to follow one nurse consistently for three hours rather than move from nurse to nurse. Also over time, I learned to nuance my requests for permission. Nurses were always thinking about their next decision, their next move, and their next task. I found I interrupted their train of thought if I consistently asked if I could follow them. My questions forced them to think about yet another decision. Instead, I became less hesitant and observed with a confidence I did not always feel.[25] Similarly, although I felt awkward keeping a distance while immersed in the situation, I tried not to offer my help with simple tasks such as getting linens or water for patients because I did not want to disrupt what I knew was a systematic process of care. For example, when I grabbed the linens to help, the nurse took time to explain where they went and reminded me to go wash my hands, because I was not wearing gloves. I became another factor to account for in her work. After each observation I wrote a log of events. I recorded physical setting, key participants, equipment used, types of physical and emotional interactions, and responses to and consequences of these interactions.

I recruited nurses for interviews over time in different ways. I introduced myself and the project repeatedly: at staff meetings, via e-mail, and on the floor. During my observation, I developed rapport with nurses in the nurses' station and in the staff room. Occasionally I ate lunch with nurses, but many nurses did not take lunch or official breaks. I specifically sought out nurses who were male, nonwhite, trained in other countries, or new. I asked permission to follow nurses on rounds and then scheduled interviews. In some cases, I scheduled interviews without observation to ensure that my sample was diverse. Some nurses approached me asking to participate; most people were comfortable with my presence and very interested in the project. Two nurses (each on a different floor) expressed concern to me. They told me they were worried about people "monitoring their work." They also said they were simply not comfortable being followed. For these nurses, I was very careful and did not intrude on their work. In all cases, I respected nurses' feelings and boundaries.

In order to understand how nurses perceive and explain intimate care in nursing, I conducted fifty-five in-depth interviews. I interviewed forty-five nurses, three nursing professors, and seven hospital administrators. The administrators included three unit directors, the director of human resources, the director of Magnet research, the vice president of clinical services, and the CEO. All administrators were white women except for the CEO, a white man.

I approached nurses for interviews while conducting my observations. I purposively sampled to obtain variance on gender, age, race, ethnicity, country of origin, and hospital unit. I asked open-ended questions in my interviews about personal background, work history, and intimate behaviors at work with patients and patients' family members.

I revised my interview schedule twice while in the field. I designed my initial interview schedule to elicit a broad range of information on multiple factors—within and outside the workplace—that affect nurses' distinctions between normal interactions in caring and intimacy in nursing from acts of harm. Informed from my initial observations, I later included questions about nurses' personal ethics and belief systems affecting care, the impact of charting and other document responsibilities, the specific impact of families, and meanings of intimacy and conflict. I conducted each interview in the setting of the participant's choice, and each lasted one to two hours. These settings included offices, coffee shops, and nurses' homes. In my interviews with administrators, I asked about how the emotional work of care affected them, staff, and the hospital at large. I also asked how the changing patient population contributed to changing nurses' work. I asked how much of nurses' work was providing care and how the hospital evaluated this work. I conducted interviews with administrators in their offices. These interviews, averaging thirty minutes, were shorter than those with nurses. I audio-recorded and transcribed each interview for analysis.

Following Robert Weiss,[26] I set a collaborative tone from the beginning of each interview to help avoid positioning myself as the "expert." As I expected, some participants generalized their responses rather than provided details. I avoided general remarks by looking for concrete instances, spoke in present tense, and inquired both about descriptions of events and about how research participants felt regarding these events. I used phrases to encourage the informant to speak (for example, "How did that start?" and "Could you walk me through it?" and "What did you mean by _____?") rather than try to anticipate what my informant would say. I returned to passing events that felt important and to let the informant lead the interview. In my first interviews in my pilot study, I noticed that I talked too much, especially by self-disclosing in an attempt to make the informant feel more comfortable. In retrospect, I realize that I felt uncomfortable and nervous. My fear of imposition was needless and if left unchecked, could have cost me opportunities to learn more about the situation I was studying.

In the tradition of qualitative research, I conducted ongoing data analysis to focus my data collection efforts. My observations focused on interactions among nurses and family members and patients, interactions between nurses and other clinical staff, and the general process of care. I typed my field notes and transcribed my interviews in Microsoft Word. I sorted and coded data along analytic themes. While some of my analyses were deductive, many categories also emerged from the data.

Throughout the project, I organized memos as discussed by Anselm L. Strauss and Juliet Corbin[27] for multiple levels of analysis: (1) code-marked notes to identify concepts to explore, (2) theory notes to develop explanations discovered in the text, and (3) operational notes for practical matters. I added "reflexive notes" to organize my own thoughts and reflections during the research process.[28] This helped me remain accountable to my own potential biases, fears, and concerns. Tracking the role of my emotions in the field and in my interviews affected my interpretations of nurses' under- standings of intimacy at work.[29] By tracking my emotions in my pilot study I found that initially I was hesitant to "hear" that nurses really did not feel sexually harassed by behaviors and interactions that I considered to constitute sexual harassment. In retrospect, I realized that my understandings of my own experiences with harassment and assault were interfering with the ways that I was analyzing these "alternative" experiences. I overcame this "block" in my thinking by writing and talking about—essentially revisiting—these experiences. Doing this work separately from my analysis helped me avoid conflating my experiences with those of my research participants.

I coded themes from my field notes and my interviews both deductively, based on those derived from my pilot project, and inductively, from analyt- ic categories that emerged in the course of my observations and interviews. Deductive codes included (1) work environment, behaviors, and definition of sexual harassment; (2) explicit discussions of sexual harassment; (3) behaviors conventionally thought of as sexual harassment, even if research participants did not define these scenarios as such, including jokes, crude remarks, and requests for sexual favors; and (4) behaviors not conventionally defined as sex- ual harassment but those that research participants defined as "inappropriate."

Inductively, I coded my notes and interviews line by line, underlined key phrases, and constructed systematic comparisons (i.e., using free lists and cognitive mapping) in order to find thematic patterns among short words or phrases. I performed in vivo coding, especially seeking categories and terms that my research participants used to describe the intimate conditions of their labor. I read my notes and interviews multiple times, back and forth, with these conditions and relations in mind and constantly asking, "When, why, and under what conditions do these themes occur in the text?" I used the condi- tional matrix as described by Strauss and Corbin[30] to check and order different levels of interactions, influences, and consequences of events. As new themes emerged, I coded and recoded these patterns and worked through remaining notes and interviews again to test these ideas. I continually checked my devel- oping ideas and explanations against competing explanations and negative cases. I adjusted my data collection to check these contrasting explanations. I used NUD*IST and NVivo software to help organize my coding efforts.

Dissemination of Findings

In January 2007, I returned to the hospital to give what Michael Burawoy calls a "valedictory visit"[31] to nurses as a part of their educational series,

Nursing Grand Rounds. I spoke on meanings of professional intimacy and how these meanings are affected by race and gender. Although I returned to provide final results to participants, not to collect more data, the visit offered opportunities for study participants to engage with me and debate the findings. As Burawoy suggests, "this is the moment of judgment, when previous relations are reassessed, theory is put to the test, and accounts are reevaluated."[32] To ensure maximum attendance, I presented in the early morning to catch nurses leaving night shift, and later in the day for day-shift workers. Nurses' responses varied. Many nurses, especially women of color, affirmed that I validated their work experiences, especially that their extra labor is taken for granted. Two administrators commented that they misunderstood the impact of nurses' and patients' race and nationality on intimate care before hearing my presentation. Most evaluations stated they wanted me to return to share more findings and they looked forward to reading the book.

It is my hope that nurses use this research to advocate for reorganization of their work space, labor, and accountability that would better accommodate professional intimacy. At the same time, I worry. Nurse administrators (even well-meaning ones) could use this data to maintain the status quo by recognizing how nurses balance professional intimacy with medical, administrative, and other care responsibilities without implementing institutional measures to support this work. Even managers who are interested in supporting professional intimate labor may inadvertently harm nurses. Managers could add to nurses' already overburdened labor by expecting nurses to formally train each other without compensation. Similarly, they could require additional charts or other documentation to standardize policies and procedures.

Ethical Concerns

As a socially responsible researcher, I continuously interrogated how my research process affected research participants and their work environments. Taking responsibility for these effects was especially important in ethnographic fieldwork because ethnography presents more opportunities for intimacy, disclosure, and feelings of familiarity between researchers and informants.[33] With this in mind, I incorporated ethical research throughout all phases of my research. I considered ethics an ongoing dialogue and set of questions and concerns specific to each new situation, rather than a problem to solve or a list of rules to check off. Rather than ask, "When do I care about my research participants?" and question the fairness of my study, I asked, "How do I appropriately care for each participant?" in each specific moment.

Ethnographers need to consider ethics in the experiences of participants as well as how we engage with these experiences. During my fieldwork and analysis, I used auto-ethnography as a mode of data collection to ensure self-reflection, my accountability, and my tracking of my own emotional work. Auto-ethnography begins with one's personal life, documents from moment to moment, and incorporates systematic introspection and emotional recall.[34] It extends beyond mere social inquiry and becomes a moral and ethical practice; it exposes vulnerabilities and subjectivities honestly and openly. For example, incorporating auto-ethnography early in my study helped me acknowledge the various contexts in which intimacy occurs at work, rather than limited my scope to meanings of sexual harassment. Conceptualizing intimacy as a process that changes over time and space helped me remain open to nurses' experiences rather than impose my own categories.

My academic and professional experience helped me consider my role as a researcher/advocate and how this role related to my work, my studies, and my interactions with hospital staff on a daily basis. Participant protection did not stop at maintaining confidentiality; it also included being sensitive to the changing workload for nurses and the subtle power dynamics between me and hospital staff, including those dynamics affected by my identity as a white woman researcher with no medical background. For example, my respect for nurses and their labor superseded any sense of entitlement to data. I was just as concerned with conforming to the norms of the field as I was with attending to any potential pitfalls from my privileged status as a white researcher in others' work environment. Many times I conformed to the environment, such as by not interacting with patients, by dutifully following nurses, by eating when others ate, and by arriving when others arrived on shift.

I continuously attended to my changing location as an "insider/outsider" in the work environment of others.[35] Although nurses' discomfort with my outsider status as researcher and student diminished as I shifted somewhat to insider status over time, my status as a medical outsider remained intact throughout the study. Some researchers who have studied the dynamics between nurses and patients are trained nurses. For example, one nurse researcher talked to me about "crossing the threshold" from researcher to caregiver when observing patients' rooms. When she conducted ethnography in a critical care unit, she provided care—for example, turning patients over in their beds or assisting with an IV.[36] I had expected that my chances to participate as observer would be diminished by my lack of medical training. This did not happen. Although I focused my efforts on cultural and social meanings of care, nurses asked me to assist them—for example, by holding equipment for them or offering a drink to a patient. I was never in a patient's room without an accompanying nurse, so when patients asked me for assistance, I deferred to the nurse. I expected to constantly negotiate my presence to avoid disruption of patient care at all costs. This was true. I negotiated the boundary between researcher and practitioner differently because I am not a trained nurse. In this way, my outsider status was an asset. However, my outsider status was not always an advantage, since it meant that I connected less to some nurses. For example, some nurses did not trust me to follow them, because they did not understand my "true" intentions. Similarly, some nurses expressed concern that human resources had hired me to evaluate them or that I spied for managers.

The intersection and level of visibility of my race, gender, sexuality, and class affected how my status switched between outsider and insider with nurses. Gaining entrée to my research site was made easier because I am white and people expect researchers to be white.[37] Since all the hospital administrators were white, I did not have to negotiate expressions of shock or disbelief, or discuss my race with them. For example, in her hospital study of Caribbean nurses, Natalie Bennett, who is Afro-Caribbean, describes repeatedly encountering initial reactions of surprise from hospital administrators and assistants who prior to meeting her had expected her to be white. In addition, Bennett's race became a topic of discussion during a meeting with unit directors to talk about how data collection would coincide with patient care. During this meeting, the vice president of nursing—a white woman—asked the other directors, directly in front of Bennett but as if she were not there, "if her being West Indian could make a difference."[38] In contrast to Bennett's experiences, my race was never a subject of discussion. No staff member or administrator seemed surprised when they learned that I was a researcher.

My race also affected interactions with nurses on the floor. I noticed that white nurses sometimes made racist remarks about patients and other nurses in front of me. On occasion, some white nurses were explicitly racist in interviews. The access my race afforded me in these situations was pronounced; these overt expressions of racism likely would not have occurred— and therefore I could not have included them in my analysis of professional intimacy—if I were not white.[39] This conjecture provides limited comfort in response to what I feel was my complicity in racism through silence. I also know that my job was to observe and understand a situation involving racism so that I could effectively address it in my writing.[40]

Most of the people of color I approached agreed to participate and seemed especially curious when they learned of my interest in race and ethnicity. This does not mean that there was no effect of race. My whiteness and my status as researcher might have afforded me privilege through what Jonathan Warren calls an "imagined superiority of whiteness" from participants.[41] Only two nurses refused to participate in my study. One nurse was African and one nurse was Caucasian. While the African nurse's decision could have resulted from racialized distrust of white women and of the research enterprise,[42] race matching does not guarantee trust.[43]

My status as a woman may have afforded me greater access to my mostly female population; however, shared gender does not always result in trust.[44] While female research participants of diverse races and ethnicities told me I was "easy to talk with," no female participant explicitly said that this was because of our shared gender. It could be that female nurses assumed, without stating, the stereotypical benefits of shared gender, in part because they were accustomed to a work environment that took female bonding for granted,[45] or it could be that our shared gender had no effect. In either case, I did not assume that my interviews with women would proceed smoothly, because shared gender can also impede conceptual development. Many times, female research participants of all races made statements such as "you know what I mean" instead of stating their meanings explicitly. This type of assumed meaning that comes from bonding, or an assumed shared experience, can lead to confused or lost meanings.[46] I paid particular attention to the potential of bonding problems with my research participants and interrupted them as they occurred. Although I usually affirmed their sentiments when bonding occurred, I also asked research participants to clarify their meanings in their own words.

When women interview men, there can also be problems specific to gender. In contrast to other reports of women interviewing men, none of the men I interviewed flirted with me, touched me, or denigrated women during the interview.[47] Early in the study, one man suggested that we meet for dinner after he got off work at 11:30 p.m. I suggested that instead we meet before his shift began. He readily agreed. The rest of my male research participants suggested I interview them at the hospital or at a public coffee shop, which meant I did not struggle with issues of safety or assumptions that we were on a "blind date."[48]

Although male nurses seemed forthright with me about their experiences of gender in nursing, my gender could have affected our interactions in other ways. Male nurses may have perceived my interviewing them as particularly threatening to their masculinity.[49] This could explain why one male nurse in particular repeatedly refused my requests for interviews. He was amiable during my observation and often volunteered his interpretations of events on the floor; thus, I opted to informally ask questions during observation. I also deferred to his experience and asked questions about acts I witnessed but did not understand.[50] I did this with all nurses, which likely helped me build rapport and avoid power conflicts. Some male research participants were minimalist at first, keeping their answers short and curt. In these cases, I referred to what other male research participants shared, for example being perceived as gay, as a way to help men feel more comfortable in the interview.[51] Male nurses may have also exaggerated their rationality, autonomy, and control when discussing their labor, as a way to preserve their masculinity, which may have altered my findings on perceptions of leadership and authority in Chapter 4.[52]

I did not calculate in advance how I would address issues of my sexuality while conducting fieldwork. Lesbianism is not new for me. I am "out of the closet" and also well aware that I often "pass" for straight. I tend not to discuss my private life in general but refer to my sexuality at work if it seems productive to do so—for example, if it contributes to teaching or to gaining research access. Because I did not foresee any benefits to disclosing my sexual identity, I decided to be noncommittal as much as possible; however, marital status can be a problem in the field.[53] I wear a wedding ring because although I am not legally married, my partner and our families and friends participated in a commitment ceremony four years ago. As far as my partner and I are concerned, we are married. Expressing concern for me in an unfamiliar city, many nurses noticed my ring and asked if my husband was in the city with me. Most often, I avoided these questions by changing the subject or just said, "I have family here." Occasionally, however, I mentioned that my partner was conducting her research or that she moved to the city partway through my study. Only a handful of times did nurses catch on and ask about my relationship or express shock that I am gay. Two nurses told me in confidence that they thought I "might be a lesbian." Although each woman identified as straight, my sexuality seemed to build rapport with them because they talked about their gay and lesbian friends and family. Although most nurses assumed I was heterosexual, I had no reason to believe that my sexuality affected my interactions with participants. I also did not know this for sure because heterosexual privilege—even gained by passing for straight—is invisible, assumed, and hard to measure.

I found that my assumed heterosexuality afforded me access to some participants. During my interview with Nadine, she expressed how some homophobic nurses on her floor care less for gay and lesbian patients. Although she emphasized her support for gay people, she admitted her discomfort with patients who were part of a lesbian couple because she did not always know how to approach them. Later, when I told her I am a lesbian, she seemed a bit embarrassed at first, but visibly relaxed when I reassured her that I was not offended by her sentiments. I found them quite important to my analysis. After this exchange, Nadine told me that another nurse would never have talked with me had he known I was gay. These comments helped me realize the impact that my perceived sexuality had on data collection efforts and the privilege I experienced because I passed for straight.[54]

I do not know if my class status as an advanced graduate student with a full-time research fellowship factored into my research. Many nurses expressed concern to me about my walking alone to my car at night in a neighborhood fraught with crime, homelessness, and drugs. These concerns could have resulted from their perceptions of my class status—that is, their perception that I had never lived in a neighborhood with a high crime rate, had never been around homeless individuals, or had not known any drug addicts and alcoholics. It was hard to tell, however, because these concerns could have stemmed from a general concern for my safety and/or could also have resulted from my white race or female gender—both of which need stereotypical protection from "dangerous" neighborhoods.

Conclusion

At first glance, my research choices seem classically feminist. For example, I chose to study the invisibility of women's work for my master's thesis, my pilot study, and my dissertation research. I was accountable to my biases about sexual harassment, and I think that my research is conceptually nuanced for it. I bridged theory and praxis by choosing a city near the Mexico border, in part because hospitals in this rapidly growing region could benefit if there were more research on these hospitals. I focused my research on the lived experiences of nurses to help nurses positively change their work environment. I prioritized the concerns of participants throughout the study and was accountable to my participants' experiences even if these participants (for example, women nurses of color) did not make up the majority of the population. I avoided disrupting the already burdensome work shifts of nurses. My data collection, analysis, and dissemination included plans that responded to the needs of my participants—as identified by the participants themselves. I obtained a sample that was diverse in race, gender, age, and ethnicity and did not rely on universal definitions of *woman*, which often means white and middle class, or of men and minorities. I hope to empower nurses as a result of my research but to do it in a way that avoids imposing extra labor on them. Did these choices make this research feminist and me a feminist researcher?

Standpoint and intersectionality theories are not in and of themselves feminist.[55] By using standpoint theory and intersectionality as methodological guides, I focused on the experiences of my participants in this research. I considered how relations of power affected public knowledge about their experiences. I listened to my research participants, even when their statements seemed antithetical to my feminist ideas. When nurses dismissed the idea of sexual harassment at work, I considered other explanations for sexualized behaviors from patients. I did not, however, always take their advice. When nurses and administrators suggested that I should not bother studying the sexual harassment of nurses by patients, I did it anyway. Similarly, I persisted in studying the impact of race even though some administrators suggested it would not be pertinent to my findings—that is, "Most nurses are white anyway."

I take social constructions of race, gender, class, ethnicity, and sexuality seriously because I know that these constructs and the intersections of these constructs have very real material and social impacts for people. Through my use of an intersectional methodology, I sampled to consider individual and group experiences of race, gender, and ethnicity. Intersectionality, as both a methodological and conceptual framework, helped me maintain my commitment to examining social and structural power dynamics in participatory research. By focusing on my identity and the impact of my presence as an outsider, I remained aware of how my identity affected my research.

These research decisions are not necessarily *only* feminist; it is true that my intentions are shared by researchers who do not identify themselves or their research as feminist. This makes my statements all the more necessary—I choose to *claim* the label of feminist for these positions. I assert feminism both to acknowledge feminist scholars' rich history doing public and activist research that cares for its participants and because naming—a historically feminist act—requires one to stake claim, to discuss, and to enter dialogue. It is in the spirit of continued dialogue that I claim my research and my researcher identity as feminist.

Appendix B

Nurse Demographics

	Female						
	Over 40 years			Under 40 years			
	U.S.	Non-U.S.	All	U.S.	Non-U.S.	All	Total
White	7 (70%)		7 (46%)	11 (73%)	3 (60%)	14 (70%)	21 (60%)
Black	3 (30%)	1 (20%)	4 (27%)	1 (7%)		1 (5%)	5 (14%)
Latina				3 (20%)	1 (20%)	4 (20%)	4 (12%)
Asian		4 (80%)	4 (27%)		1 (20%)	1 (5%)	5 (14%)
Total	10	5	15	15	5	20	35

	Male						
	Over 40 years			Under 40 years			
	U.S.	Non-U.S.	All	U.S.	Non-U.S.	All	Total
White	3 (75%)			5 (83%)			8 (80%)
Nonwhite	1 (25%)			1 (17%)			2 (20%)
Total	4			6			10

Appendix C

Illustrations: Model of Professional Intimacy and Nursing School Recruitment

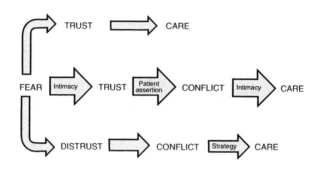

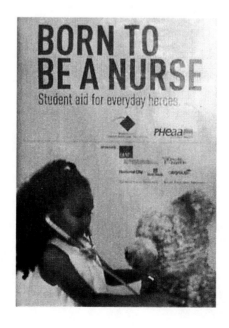

Notes

INTRODUCTION

1. All names are pseudonyms. Anna is a nurse in my study. What follows is based on my observations of her and my interviews with her.

2. Scherzer 2003.

3. Glazer 1991; Hine 1989; Melosh 1982; Reverby 1987; Scherzer 2003.

4. Duffy 2007; Nakano Glenn 2002.

5. Collins 2000; Nakano Glenn 2002, 2010.

6. Choy 2003.

7. Davies 1996.

8. Gordon 2005 discusses this, too.

9. Zelizer 2005.

10. For accounts in nursing scholarship that claim the importance of intimacy from the perspective of the bedside nurse but also call for more research to examine its complexity, see Dowling 2003, 2006; Kadner 1994; Kirk 2007; Nikkonen 1994; Savage 1995; and A. Williams 2001a, 2001b. I should also note that the relationship between negotiating intimacy and negotiating conflict is not part of any of these accounts. For an article that challenges this claim, see Allan 2002.

11. Perrin 2007; Shattell 2004.

12. Dowling 2008 also describes "nurse-patient intimacy" as a process in oncology nursing. Dowling reports that nurses negotiate a "professional friend" role that helps maintain the nurse's empathy for and identification with the patient. Dowling explains that patients influence the relationship with nurses, especially because the patient's individual characteristics contribute to how nurses can identify with their patients. Just as I advocate for collective intimate practices later in this book, Dowling claims that "peer support" helps nurses conduct and maintain intimacy with their individual patients.

13. This could also result from nurses' discomfort working with and around bodies. See Picco, Santoro, and Garrino 2010.

14. For a look at one study that examines the relationship between intimacy in nursing care and patient-preferred gender of the nurse, see Chur-Hansen 2002.

15. Additional information on my method can be found in Appendix A.

16. Collins 1999, 2000; Crenshaw 1989, 1991, 1992.

17. I discuss standpoint theory further in Appendix A.

18. Anderson, Leonard, and Yates 1974.

19. Zelizer 2005.

20. In nursing scholarship, this dynamic has been referred to as negotiating a balance between distance and intimacy. See Allan and Barber 2005.

21. Collins 2000; Duffy 2005; Hondagneu-Sotelo 2001; Nakano Glenn 2002, 2010.

22. Das Gupta 2009; Hine 1989; Scherzer 2003.

23. I am both committed to and cautious about my choice to use the phrase *women of color* in this book. I am committed to the phrase because it helps to identify significant patterns in experiences faced by women who are not white and share similar forms of discrimination and possibilities for solidarity based on how others perceive their skin tone. My use of the phrase *of color* also recognizes that skin color is a powerful component in practices of racism, xenophobia, and white privilege. For example, in her renowned book, *Black Feminist Thought*, Patricia Hill Collins (2000) identifies the power of colorism as a by-product of racism. Specifically, Collins changes the conversation on beauty discrimination by introducing the power of skin tone as it negotiates systemic opportunity and privilege for black women. Finally, I first learned about the phrase *women of color* when reading scholarly writings by multicultural feminists and since have used this terminology to highlight the agency and power of women of color, rather than focusing only on oppression. I am cautious about my use of the phrase because too often phrases like this one and others such as *third-world women* become static and are used as universal descriptors for women across nation, culture, and race who are very different. See two classic articles that discuss the pitfalls of monolithic language to describe women who are diverse by race and nation: Dill 1983 and Mohanty 2002.

24. Ehrenreich and Hochschild 2002.

25. C. Williams 1993, 1995.

26. C. Williams 1995.

27. Harvey Wingfield 2009.

28. Crenshaw 1992: 1473.

29. Crenshaw 1989, 1992.

30. Beiner 2005.

31. Collins 1999 and a presentation by Kimberlé Crenshaw and Bonnie Thornton Dill at the 2009 National Women Studies Association meeting in Atlanta, Georgia.

32. Berger and Guidroz 2010.

33. Boris and Parrenas 2010.

34. Zelizer 2010.

35. Zelizer 2009, 2010.

36. Zelizer 2010: 278.

37. Ibid.

38. B. Anderson 2000; Barton 2006; Price-Glynn 2010; Hondagneu-Sotelo 2001; Ehrenreich and Hochschild 2002.

39. Dellinger and Williams 2002; Guiffre and Williams 1994; Hoffman 2004; Lerum 2004.

40. Owings 2002; Huebner 1994; Cobble 1991.

41. Gordon 2005 includes a useful analysis of how media representations of sexy nurses negatively affect the work conditions of real nurses.

42. Bronner 2003; Hanrahan 1997; Libbus and Bowman 1994; C. Williams 1995.

43. In Chapter 2, I discuss Miliann Kang's work in more detail, notably how she extends Hochschild's concept of emotional labor to coin and conceptualize body labor.

44. Hochschild 1983.

45. Ibid., 147.

46. Bolton 2000.

47. Bolton and Boyd 2003; Lopez 2006.

48. James 1989, 1992.

49. Henderson 2001.

50. Bolton 2001.

51. Parrenas 2005.

52. Boris and Parrenas 2010.

53. Kingma 2006.

54. Zelizer 2005.

55. Ibid., 187.

56. Ibid., 153.

57. Gordon 2005.

58. Nelson 2004; Nelson and Gordon 2006; Watson 2003, 2005.

59. Nelson and Gordon 2006.

CHAPTER 1

1. Retrieved from the hospital's website, May 19, 2010.

2. Here I draw from various ideas and ideologies that challenge the idea that intimacy is about only one's personal sexuality. Sociologist Viviana Zelizer (2005) argues that intimacy is not just personal and must be recognized for its social and economic functions. I also consider how Michel Foucault (1980) helps us think about how our failure to discuss intimacy in public life comes, in part, from our fear of stigma. Finally, I think about what sociologist Bernadette Barton (2006) calls the feminist sex wars. Nurses may be afraid to talk about intimacy because they want to avoid being labeled as either a victim of sexual objectification or a proponent of sexual freedom.

3. These and similar comments were made by nurses, nurse administrators, and educators.

4. Gordon 2005.

5. Ibid., 157.

6. Reverby 1987.

7. Welter 1966.

8. Rothenberg 2002.

9. Gordon 2005.

10. Whittock and Leonard 2003.

11. Collins 2000; Hondagneu-Sotelo 2001; Ehrenreich and Hochschild 2002; Nakano Glenn 2002.

12. Dill 1983.

13. Duffy 2007; Nakano Glenn 2002.

14. Duffy 2005.

15. Duffy 2005; Nakano Glenn 2002; Scherzer 2003.

16. C. Williams 1995. But as Harvey Wingfield (2009) notes, this does not necessarily include male nurses of color.

17. Harvey Wingfield (2009) also found this in her study of black men in nursing.

18. Connell 1995: 45.

19. Connell 1995.

20. West and Zimmerman 1987.

21. Connell 1995.

22. Connell 2001.

23. Pharr 1988.

24. Davies 1996.

25. Here I refer to an advertisement produced by the Oregon Center for Nursing with a headline that reads, "Are you man enough to be a nurse?" Pictured are several men standing in traditionally masculine poses with their arms crossed over their chests and their feet set apart. Each man is either wearing nurses' scrubs or traditionally masculine clothing such as a business suit, T-shirt and jeans, and a karate uniform. One man is holding a football. No one is smiling.

26. Connell 1987.

27. Abbott 1998; Melosh 1982. Also, the idea of a true woman is rooted in "the cult of true womanhood" discussed in this chapter.

28. Ehrenreich and Hochschild 2002; Hochschild 1983; Misra 2003.

29. Bolton and Boyd 2003.

30. Kittay and Feder 2002; Meyer 2000.

31. Bolton 2000.

32. Gordon 2005.

33. Reverby 1987.

34. Nelson 2003.

35. Nelson and Gordon 2006.

36. Watson 2003, 2005.

37. Wolf 1988.

38. Nelson 2004.

39. Nelson and Gordon 2006.

40. Davies 1996; Gordon 2005; Melosh 1982; Nelson and Gordon 2006; Reverby 1987.

41. Davies 1996.

42. Woodward 1997.

43. Weinburg 2003.

44. Frye 1983.

45. Field notes, July 2005.

46. Collins 2000.

47. Savage 1987.

48. Bronner, Peretz, and Ehrenfeld 2003; Hanrahan 1997; Libbus and Bowman 1994; C. Williams 1995.

49. Fiedler and Hamby 2000; Neuhs 1994.

50. McGuire, Dougherty, and Atkinson 2006.

51. Dowling 2003 and Kirk 2007 also discuss the likelihood that nurses' discomfort with the word *intimacy* comes from the term's common association with sexuality.

52. Kittay and Feder 2002.

53. Huebner 2008; see also Hanrahan 1997.

54. Hellzen et al. 2004.

55. Benner 1984.

56. Padgett 2000.

57. Shapiro 1998.

58. Bradshaw 2001.

59. May and Veitch 1998.

60. Carryer, Russell, and Budge 2007.

61. Nelson 2004.

62. Goodman 2007.

63. Baltimore 2004; Dracup 2004.

64. Swanson 1991.

65. Jacobs 2001; Gastmans 1999.

66. Nelson and McGillion 2004; Padgett 2000.

67. Field notes, October 2005.

CHAPTER 2

1. Field notes, December 2005.

2. Ehrenreich and Hochschild 2002; Folbre 2001; Hochschild 1983, 2000; Kang 2003; Misra 2003.

3. Gordon 2005; Davies 1996.

4. Abbott 1998; Melosh 1982.

5. Crenshaw 1989.

6. Moraga and Anzaldua 1979.

7. B. Smith 1983.

8. Davis 1981; Lorde 1984.

9. Anzaldua 1987.

10. Mohanty 2002.

11. See Berger and Guidroz 2010 (especially the conversation among Kimberlé Crenshaw, Michele Fine, and Nira Yuval-Davis) for details. One concern in particular is how intersectionality is used to justify a "flattening" effect. To flatten social experiences (or scientific data) means to only describe multiple identities rather than analyze how identity location is systematically affected by structural power. In the same anthology, Ann Russo discusses the problem of simply giving a nod to intersectionality. She details how Gloria Steinem failed to analyze the 2008 presidential race as one of race-gender. She named intersectionality but then returned to making gender the primary salient category in her analysis.

12. Rothenberg 2002.

13. Spelman 1988.

14. McCall 2005; Welsh et al. 2006.

15. Collins 1999.

16. Ibid., 268.

17. Anderson 2000; Boris and Parrenas 2010; Nakano Glenn 2002; Hondagneu-Sotelo 2001; Kang 2003, 2010.

18. Berger and Guidroz 2010.

19. Ibid., 7.

20. Field notes, December 2005.

21. 2000: 72.

22. Choy 2003.

23. Duffy 2007; Nakano Glenn 2002.

24. McCall 2005.

25. Kingma 2006 and my field notes.

26. Hochschild 2000, 2003.

27. Weinburg 2003.

28. Hochschild 2000; Moody 1997.

29. Ehrenreich and Hochschild 2002; Folbre 2001; Hochschild 1983, 2000; Kang 2003; Misra 2003; Sassen 2002.

30. Kingma 2006.

31. Ehrenreich and Hochschild 2002.

32. Kingma 2006.

33. Satterly 2004.

34. The hospital I studied was a Magnet hospital that also relied on immigrant nurses.

35. Choy 2003.

36. Buchan and Calman 2004.

37. Weinburg 2003.

38. Gordon 2005.

39. Coordinating patient care is described in the hospital's job posts as "coordinates patient care, team activities and plan of care with other healthcare team members." The nurses I interviewed and observed freely used the term "coordinate" to discuss balancing the responsibility.

40. The comment was made by Jody, a white, female experienced nurse.

41. Bolton 2000.

42. Hochschild 1983; Kang 2010.

43. Kang 2010. It is also noteworthy that Kang frames her concept of body labor as an extension of emotional labor.

44. Field notes, January 2005.

45. 2000: 70.

46. Ibid., 71.

47. Quoted from an interview with the vice president of clinical care.

48. Nurses report that they would rather spend more time with patients, but they are required to spend extensive time on their charting (Gordon 2005; Weinburg 2003). As nurses try to balance patient care with institutional demands, they experience a time bind because there is simply not enough time to accomplish all tasks (Hochschild 1997).

CHAPTER 3

1. Faugier 2006.
2. Zerubavel 2006.
3. Rothenberg 2002.
4. Nakano Glenn (2002) explains the historical roots of this pattern that I see in nursing.
5. Collins 2000.
6. Nakano Glenn 2002.
7. Chang 2000.
8. At the time of this writing, Arizona has passed anti-immigration Senate Bill 1070, and replicate strategies are quickly picking up speed. Lawmakers in New York, Washington, Nevada, and Rhode Island are reporting plans to introduce new legislation that increases border security and/or requires anyone to carry citizenship documents on their person. Currently, Arizona Senate Bill 1070 requires police to detain anyone they "reasonably" suspect of illegal immigration; police do not need a warrant to stop or arrest anyone they suspect of undocumented citizenship status. This puts Arizona Latinos and Latinas at serious risk for racial profiling.
9. Choy 2003; Takahashi 2004.
10. Zelizer 2005.

CHAPTER 4

1. Collins 2000.
2. Ibid.
3. Kang 2010: 5.
4. I first found this pattern in my pilot study with nurses in a large hospital in Pittsburgh, Pennsylvania. See Huebner 2008 for more information.
5. Gordon 2005.
6. Anderson 2000.

CHAPTER 5

1. See Hem and Heggen 2003 for an explicit discussion of the need for more research on the necessary balance between intimacy and distance for nurses who work with psychiatric patients.
2. Frye 1983.
3. It may not be a coincidence that Patsy is an immigrant nurse trained in Canada. In many of our conversations, she noted the difference between her training in Canada, which included a greater focus on collaborative nursing, and her work experience in the United States.

CONCLUSION

1. My intention is to focus on systematic and visible patterns, not on individual nurses' care work. Many individual nurses in my study cared for patients extremely well

in spite of this fact. The hospital I studied was a nursing Magnet hospital, which means that it was in the top 2 percent of the country for best nursing practices.

APPENDIX A

1. Studying Naples 2003 helped me immensely in my consideration of the parameters involved in this definition.
2. D. Smith 2005.
3. Stacey 1988.
4. Blee 2000.
5. D. Smith 1997.
6. Collins 1999.
7. See also Giuffre and Williams 1994 and Hanrahan 1997.
8. Huebner 2008.
9. Huebner 2005.
10. Clawson 2003.
11. Burawoy 2000.
12. Harding 1997; Hartsock 1997; D. Smith 1997.
13. D. Smith 1987, 1990.
14. Hartsock 1983, 1985.
15. Collins 2000; hooks 1984.
16. Blee 2000 and conversation with Kathleen Blee in 2005.
17. Rothenberg 2002.
18. Collins 1999.
19. Twine 2000.
20. Conversation with Cecila Green during a 2005 lecture given by Nancy Naples at the University of Pittsburgh.
21. Happ 1998.
22. Garfinkel 1967.
23. Becker 1993.
24. Richardson 2003; Blee 1998.
25. Becker 1993.
26. Weiss 1994.
27. Strauss and Corbin 1990.
28. Richardson 2003.
29. Blee 1998.
30. 1990.
31. Burawoy 2003: 672.
32. Ibid.
33. Stacey 1988.
34. Richardson 2003.
35. Collins 1986.
36. Happ 1998.
37. Warren 2000.
38. Bennett 2002: 107.
39. Blee 2000.

40. Becker 2000.
41. 2000: 161.
42. Zinn 1979, 1990.
43. Twine 2000.
44. Riessman 1987.
45. Dellinger and Williams 2002.
46. Blee 1998; Schwalbe and Wolkomir 2001.
47. Arendell 1997; Lee 1997.
48. Arendell 1997; Lee 1997.
49. Schwalbe and Wolkomir 2001.
50. Ibid.
51. Arendell 1997; Lee 1997.
52. Arendell 1997; Lee 1997.
53. Lewin and Leap 1996.
54. Goodman 1996.
55. D. Smith 1997.

References

Abbott, Pamela. 1998. *The Sociology of the Caring Professions*. Philadelphia: UCL Press.

Allan, Helen T. 2002. "Nursing the Clinic, Being There and Hovering: Ways of Caring in a British Fertility Unit." *Journal of Advanced Nursing* 38 (1): 86–93.

Allan, Helen T., and Debbie Barber. 2005. "Emotional Boundary Work in Advanced Fertility Nursing Roles." *Nursing Ethics* 12 (4): 391–400.

Anderson, Bridget. 2000. *Doing the Dirty Work: The Global Politics of Domestic Labour*. New York: Zed Books.

Anderson, Eva Mae, Barbara J. Leonard, and Judith A. Yates. 1974. "Epigenesis of the Nurse Practitioner Role." *American Journal of Nursing* 74 (10): 1812–1816.

Anzaluda, Gloria. 1987. *Borderlands/La Frontera: The New Mestiza*. San Francisco, CA: Aunt Lute Books.

Arendell, Terry. 1997. "Reflections on the Researcher-Researched Relationship: A Woman Interviewing Men." *Qualitative Sociology* 20:341–368.

Baltimore, Jane J. 2004. "The Hospital Clinical Preceptor: Essential Preparation for Success." *Journal of Continuing Education in Nursing* 35:133–140.

Barton, Bernadette. 2006. *Stripped: Inside the Lives of Exotic Dancers*. New York: New York University Press.

Becker, Howard. 1993. "How I Learned What a Crock Was." *Journal of Contemporary Ethnography* 22:28–35.

———. 2000. "Afterword: Racism and the Research Process." In *Racing Research, Researching Race: Methodological Dilemmas in Critical Race Studies*, edited by France Winddance Twine and Jonathan W. Warren, 247–253. New York: New York University Press.

Beiner, Theresa. 2005. *Gender Myths vs. Working Realities: Using Social Science to Reformulate Sexual Harassment Law*. New York: New York University Press.

Benner, Patricia. 1984. *From Novice to Expert: Excellence and Power in Clinical Nursing Practice.* Menlo Park, CA: Addison-Wesley.

Bennett, Natalie D. A. 2002. "Work Makes a Woman? Gender, Ethnicity and Work in Afro-Caribbean Immigrant Women's Lives." Ph.D. diss., University of Michigan.

Berger, Michelle Tracey, and Kathleen Guidroz, eds. 2010. *The Intersectional Approach: Transforming the Academy through Race, Class, and Gender.* Chapel Hill: University of North Carolina Press.

Blee, Kathleen M. 1998. "White-Knuckle Research: Emotional Dynamics in Fieldwork with Racist Activists." *Qualitative Sociology* 21:381–399.

———. 2000. "White on White: Interviewing Women in U.S. White Supremacist Groups." In *Racing Research, Researching Race: Methodological Dilemmas in Critical Race Studies,* edited by France Winddance Twine and Jonathan W. Warren, 93–111. New York: New York University Press.

Bolton, Sharon C. 2000. "Who Cares? Offering Emotion Work as a 'Gift' in the Nursing Labour Process." *Journal of Advanced Nursing* 32:580–586.

———. 2001. "Changing Faces: Nurses as Emotional Jugglers." *Sociology of Health and Illness* 23:85–100.

Bolton, Sharon, and Carol Boyd. 2003. "Trolly Dolly or Skilled Emotion Manager? Moving on from Hochschild's Managed Heart." *Work, Employment and Society* 17:289–308.

Boris, Eileen, and Rhacel Salazar Parrenas, eds. 2010. *Intimate Labors: Cultures, Technologies, and the Politics of Care.* Palo Alto, CA: Stanford University Press.

Bradshaw, Ann. 2001. *The Project 2000 Nurses: The Remaking of British General Nursing 1978–2000.* London: Whurr Publishers.

Bronner, Gila, Chava Peretz, and Mally Ehrenfeld. 2003. "Sexual Harassment of Nurses and Nursing Students." *Journal of Advanced Nursing* 42:637–644.

Buchan, James, and Lynn Calman. 2004. *The Global Shortage of Registered Nurses: An Overview of Issues and Actions.* Geneva, Switzerland: International Council of Nurses.

Burawoy, Michael. 2000. *Global Ethnography: Forces, Connections, and Imaginations in the Modern World.* Berkeley: University of California Press.

———. 2003. "Revisits: An Outline of a Theory of Reflexive Ethnography." *American Sociological Review* 68 (5): 645–678.

Carryer, Jenny, Anne Russell, and Claire Budge. 2007. "Nurses' Understanding of the Professional Development Recognition Programme." *Nursing Praxis in New Zealand* 23:5–13.

Chang, Grace. 2000. *Disposable Domestics: Immigrant Women Workers in the Global Economy.* Cambridge, MA: South End Press.

Choy, Catherine Ceniza. 2003. *Empire of Care: Nursing and Migration in Filipino American History.* Durham, NC: Duke University Press.

Chur-Hansen, Anna. 2002. "Preferences for Female and Male Nurses: The Role of Age, Gender, and Previous Experience—Year 2000 Compared with 1984." *Journal of Advanced Nursing* 37 (2): 192–198.

Clawson, Dan. 2003. *The Next Upsurge: Labor and the New Social Movements.* Ithaca, NY: ILR Press.

Cobble, Dorothy Sue. 1991. *Dishing It Out.* Urbana: University of Illinois Press.

Collins, Patricia Hill. 1986. "Learning from the Outsider Within: The Sociological Significance of Black Feminist Thought." *Social Problems* 33:14–32.

———. 1999. "Moving beyond Gender: Intersectionality and Scientific Knowledge." In *Revisioning Gender*, edited by Myra Marx Ferree, Judith Lorber, and Beth B. Hess, 261–284. Thousand Oaks, CA: Sage.

———. 2000. *Black Feminist Thought: Knowledge, Consciousness, and the Politics of Empowerment.* 2nd ed. New York: Routledge.

Connell, Raewyn. 1987. *Gender and Power: Society, the Person, and Sexual Politics.* Palo Alto, CA: Stanford University Press.

———. 1995. *Masculinities.* Berkeley: University of California Press.

———. 2001. *The Men and the Boys.* Berkeley: University of California Press.

Crenshaw, Kimberlé. 1989. "Demarginalizing the Intersection of Race and Sex: A Black Feminist Critique of Antidiscrimination Doctrine, Feminist Theory and Antiracist Politics." University of Chicago Legal Forum.

———. 1991. "Mapping the Margins: Intersectionality, Identity Politics, and Violence against Women of Color." *Stanford Law Review* 43:1241–1299.

———. 1992. "Race, Gender, and Sexual Harassment." *Southern California Law Review* 65:1467–1476.

Das Gupta, Tania. 2009. *Real Nurses and Others: Racism in Nursing.* Winnipeg, Canada: Fernwood Publishing.

Davies, Celia. 1996. *Gender and the Professional Predicament in Nursing.* Buckingham, UK: OU Press.

Davis, Angela Y. 1981. *Women, Race and Class.* New York: Vintage.

Dellinger, Kirstin, and Christine Williams. 2002. "The Locker Room and the Dorm Room: Workplace Norms and the Boundaries of Sexual Harassment in Magazine Editing." *Social Problems* 49:242–257.

Dill, Bonnie Thornton. 1983. "Race, Class, and Gender: Prospects for an All-Inclusive Sisterhood." *Feminist Studies* 9 (1): 131–150.

Dowling, Maura. 2003. A Concept Analysis of Intimacy in Nursing. *All Ireland Journal of Nursing and Midwifery* 2 (11): 40–46.

———. 2006. "The Sociology of Intimacy in the Nurse-Patient Relationship. *Nursing Standard* 20 (23): 48–54.

———. 2008. "The Meaning of Nurse-Patient Intimacy in Oncology Care Settings: From the Nurse and Patient Perspective." *European Journal of Oncology Nursing* 12 (4): 319–328.

Dracup, Kathleen. 2004. "From Novice to Expert to Mentor: Shaping the Future of Nursing. *American Journal of Critical Care* 13:448–450.

Duffy, Mignon. 2005. "Reproducing Labor Inequalities: Challenges for Feminists Conceptualizing Care at the Intersections of Gender, Race, and Class." *Gender and Society* 19 (1): 66–82.

———. 2007. "Doing the Dirty Work: Gender, Race, and Reproductive Labor in Historical Perspective." *Gender and Society* 21 (3): 313–336.

Ehrenreich, Barbara, and Arlie Russell Hochschild. 2002. *Global Woman: Nannies, Maids, and Sex Workers in the New Economy.* New York: Metropolitan Books.

Faugier, Jean. 2006. "Intimacy in Nursing." *Nursing Standard* 20 (52): 20–22.

Fiedler, Anne, and Eileen Hamby. 2000. "Sexual Harassment in the Workplace: Nurses' Perceptions." *Journal of Nursing Administrators* 30:497–503.

Folbre, Nancy. 2001. *The Invisible Heart: Economics and Family Values.* New York: New Press.

Foucault, Michel. 1980. *The History of Sexuality, Volume I: An Introduction*. New York: Vintage.

Frye, Marilyn. 1983. *The Politics of Reality: Essays in Feminist Theory*. Freedom, CA: Crossing Press.

Garfinkel, Harold. 1967. *Studies in Ethnomethodology*. Englewood Cliffs, NJ: Prentice Hall.

Gastmans, Chris. 1999. "Care as a Moral Attitude in Nursing." *Nursing Ethics* 6:214–223.

Giuffre, Patti A., and Christine L. Williams. 1994. "Boundary Lines: Labeling Sexual Harassment in Restaurants." *Gender and Society* 8:378–401.

Glazer, Nona. 1991. "Between a Rock and a Hard Place: Women's Professional Organizations in Nursing and Class, Racial, and Ethnic Inequalities." *Gender and Society* 5:351–372.

Goodman, Benny. 2007. "Rules of Engagement." *Nursing Standard* 28:61.

Goodman, Liz. 1996. "Rites of Passing." In *Out in the Field: Reflections of Lesbian and Gay Anthropologists*, edited by Ellen Lewin and William Leap, 49–57. Chicago: University of Illinois Press.

Gordon, Suzanne. 2005. *Nursing against the Odds: How Health Care Cost Cutting, Media Stereotypes, and Medical Hubris Undermine Nurses and Patient Care*. Ithaca, NY: ILR Press of Cornell University Press.

Hanrahan, Patricia M. 1997. "How Do I Know If I'm Being Harassed or If This Is a Part of My Job? Nurses and Definitions of Sexual Harassment." *NWSA Journal* 9:43–64.

Happ, Mary Beth. 1998. "A Grounded Theory Study of Treatment Interference in Critically Ill Adults." Ph.D. diss., University of Pennsylvania.

Harding, Sandra. 1997. "Comment on Hekman's 'Truth and Method: Feminist Standpoint Theory Revisited.'" *Signs* 22:382–392.

Hartsock, Nancy. 1983. "The Feminist Standpoint: Developing the Ground for a Specifically Feminist Historical Materials." In *Discovering Reality*, edited by S. Harding and M. B. Hinktikka, 283–310. Amsterdam: D. Reidel.

———. 1985. *Money, Sex, and Power: Towards a Feminist Historical Materialism*. Boston: Northeastern University Press.

———. 1997. "Comment on Hekman's 'Truth and Method: Feminist Standpoint Theory Revisited.'" *Signs* 22:367–375.

Harvey Wingfield, Adia. 2009. "Racializing the Glass Escalator: Reconsidering Men's Experiences with Women's Work." *Gender and Society* 23 (1): 5–26.

Hellzen, Ove, Kenneth Asplund, Per-Olof Sandman, and Astrid Norberg. 2004. "The Meaning of Caring as Described by Nurses Caring for a Person Who Acts Provokingly: An Interview Study." *Scandinavian Journal of Caring Sciences* 18:3–11.

Hem, Marit Helene, and Kristin Heggen. 2003. "Being Professional and Being Human: One Nurse's Relationship with a Psychiatric Patient." *Journal of Advanced Nursing* 43 (1): 101–108.

Henderson, Angela. 2001. "Emotional Labor and Nursing: An Under-appreciated Aspect of Caring Work." *Nursing Inquiry* 8:130–138.

Hine, Darlene Clark. 1989. *Black Women in White: Racial Conflict and Cooperation in the Nursing Profession, 1890–1950*. Bloomington: University of Indiana Press.

Hochschild, Arlie Russell. 1983. *The Managed Heart: Commercialization of Human Feeling*. Berkeley: University of California Press.

————. 1997. *The Time-Bind: When Work Becomes Home and Home Becomes Work*. New York: Henry Holt.

————. 2000. "Global Care Chains and Emotional Surplus Value." In *On the Edge: Living with Global Capitalism*, edited by Will Hutton and Anthony Giddens, 130–146. London: Jonathan Cape.

Hoffman, Elizabeth. 2004. "Selective Sexual Harassment: Differential Treatment of Similar Groups of Women Workers." *Law and Human Behavior* 28:29–45.

Hondagneu-Sotelo, Pierrette. 2001. *Domestica: Immigrant Workers Cleaning and Caring in the Shadows of Affluence*. Berkeley: University of California Press.

hooks, bell. 1984. *Ain't I a Woman: Black Women and Feminism*. Boston: South End Press.

Huebner, Lisa C. 1994. "Sexual Harassment in Waitress Positions: An Examination of Victims' Perceptions," M.A. thesis, University of Cincinnati.

————. 2008. "It Is Part of the Job: Waitresses and Nurses Define Sexual Harassment." *Sociological Viewpoints* (Fall): 75–90.

Jacobs, Barbara Bennett. 2001. "Respect for Human Dignity: A Central Phenomenon to Philosophically Unite Nursing Theory and Practice through Consilience of Knowledge." *Advanced Nursing Science* 24:17–35.

James, Nicky. 1989. Emotional Labour: Skill and Work in the Social Regulation of Feeling." *Sociological Review* 37:15–42.

————. 1992. "Care = Organisation + Physical Labour + Emotional Labour." *Sociology of Health and Illness* 14:488–509.

Kadner, Kathleen. 1994. "Therapeutic Intimacy in Nursing." *Journal of Advanced Nursing* 19:215–218.

Kang, Miliann. 2003. "The Managed Hand: The Commercialization of Bodies and Emotions in Korean Immigrant-Owned Nail Salons." *Gender and Society* 17:820–839.

————. 2010. *The Managed Hand: Race, Gender, and the Body in Beauty Service Work*. Berkeley: University of California Press.

Kingma, Mireille. 2006. *Nurses on the Move: Migration and the Global Health Care Economy*. Ithaca, NY: ILR Press of Cornell University Press.

Kirk, Timothy W. 2007. "Beyond Empathy: Clinical Intimacy in Nursing Practice." *Nursing Philosophy* 8:233–243.

Kittay, Eva Feder, and Ellen K. Feder. 2002. *The Subject of Care: Feminist Perspectives on Dependency*. New York: Rowman and Littlefield.

Lee, Deborah. 1997. "Interviewing Men: Vulnerabilities and Dilemmas." *Women's Studies International Forum* 20 (4): 553–564.

Lerum, Kari. 2004. "Sexuality, Power, and Camaraderie in Service Work." *Gender and Society* 18:756–776.

Lewin, Ellen, and William Leap, eds.1996. *Out in the Field: Reflections of Lesbian and Gay Anthropologists*. Chicago: University of Illinois Press.

Libbus, M. Kay, and Katherine G. Bowman. 1994. "Sexual Harassment of Female Registered Nurses in Hospitals." *Journal of Nursing Administrators* 24:26–31.

Lopez, Steven. 2006. "Emotional Labor and Organized Emotional Care: Conceptualizing Nursing Home Care Work." *Work and Occupations* 33:133–160.

Lorde, Audre. 1984. "Age, Race, Class, and Sex: Women Redefining Difference." *Sister Outsider.* Freedom, CA: Crossing Press.

May, Nick, and Lin Veitch. 1998. "Working to Learn and Learning to Work: Placement Experiences of Project 2000 Nursing Students in Scotland." *Nurse Education Today* 18:630–636.

McCall, Leslie. 2005. "The Complexity of Intersectionality." *Signs: Journal of Women in Culture and Society* 30:1771–1800.

McGuire, Tammy, Debbie S. Dougherty, and Joshua Atkinson. 2006. "Paradoxing the Dialectic: The Impact of Patients' Sexual Harassment in the Discursive Construction of Nurses' Caregiving Roles." *Management Communication Quarterly* 19:416–450.

Melosh, Barbara. 1982. *The Physician's Hand: Work Culture and Conflict in American Nursing.* Philadelphia: Temple University Press.

Meyer, Madonna Harrington. 2000. *Care Work: Gender, Class, and the Welfare State.* New York: Routledge.

Misra, Joya. 2003. "Caring about Care." *Feminist Studies* 29:387–401.

Mohanty, Chandra Talpade. 2002. "Under Western Eyes Revisited: Feminist Solidarity through Anticapitalist Struggles." *Signs* 28 (2): 499–535.

Moody, Kim. 1997. *Workers in a Lean World: Unions in the International Economy.* London: Verso Press.

Moraga, Cherríe, and Gloria Anzaldua. 1979. *This Bridge Called My Back: Writings by Radical Women of Color.* Latham, NY: Kitchen Table Women of Color Press.

Nakano Glenn, Evelyn. 2002. *Unequal Freedom: How Race and Gender Shaped American Citizenship and Labor.* Cambridge, MA: Harvard University Press.

———. 2010. *Forced to Care: Coercion and Care Giving in America.* Cambridge, MA: Harvard University Press.

Naples, Nancy. 2003. *Feminism and Method: Ethnography, Discourse Analysis, and Activist Research.* New York: Routledge.

Nelson, Sioban. 2003. *Say Little, Do Much: Nursing, Nuns, and Hospitals in the 19th Century.* Philadelphia: University of Pennsylvania Press.

———. 2004. "The Search for Good in Nursing? The Burden of Ethical Expertise." *Nursing Philosophy* 5:12–22.

Nelson, Sioban, and Suzanne Gordon. 2006. "Moving beyond the Virtue Script in Nursing." In *The Complexities of Care: Nursing Reconsidered,* edited by Sioban Nelson and Suzanne Gordon, 1–12. Ithaca, NY: Cornell University Press.

Nelson, Sioban, and Michael McGillion. 2004. "Expertise or Performance? Questioning the Rhetoric of Contemporary Narrative Use in Nursing." *Journal of Advanced Nursing* 47:631–638.

Neuhs, Helen P. 1994. "Sexual Harassment: A Concern for Nursing Administrators." *Journal of Nursing Administrators* 24:47–52.

Nikkonen, Merja. 1994. "Caring from the Point of View of a Finnish Mental Health Nurse: A Life History Approach." *Journal of Advanced Nursing* 19:1185–1195.

Owings, Allison. 2002. *Hey Waitress! The USA from the Other Side of the Tray.* Berkeley: University of California Press.

Padgett, Stephen M. 2000. "Benner and the Critics: Promoting Scholarly Dialogue." *Scholarly Inquiry for Nursing Practice* 14:249–266.

Parrenas, Rhacel Salazar. 2005. *Children of Global Migration: Transnational Families and Gendered Woes.* Palo Alto, CA: Stanford University Press.

Perrin, Kathleen O. 2007. *Quick Look Nursing: Ethics and Conflict.* Burlington, MA: Jones and Bartlett.

Pharr, Suzanne. 1988. *Homophobia: A Weapon of Sexism.* Little Rock, AR: Chardon Press.

Picco, Elisa, Roberto Santoro, and Lorenza Garrino. 2010. "Dealing with the Patient's Body in Nursing: Nurses' Ambiguous Experience in Clinical Practice." *Nursing Inquiry* 17 (1): 39–46.

Price-Glynn, Kim. 2010. *Strip Club: Gender, Power, and Sex Work.* New York: New York University Press.

Reverby, Susan M. 1987. *Ordered to Care: The Dilemma of American Nursing, 1850–1945.* New York: Cambridge University Press.

Richardson, Laurel. 2003. "Writing: A Method of Inquiry." In *Collecting and Interpreting Qualitative Materials,* edited by Norman K. Denzin and Yvonne S. Lincoln, 441–499. Thousand Oaks, CA: Sage.

Riessman, Catherine Kohler. 1987. "When Gender Is Not Enough: Women Interviewing Women." *Gender and Society* 1:172–207.

Rothenberg, Paula S. 2002. *White Privilege: Essential Readings on the Other Side of Racism.* New York: Worth Publishers.

Sassen, Saskia. 2002. "Global Cities and Survival Circuits." In *Global Woman: Nannies, Maids, and Sex Workers in the New Economy,* edited by Barbara Ehrenreich and Arlie Russell Hochschild, 254–274. New York: Metropolitan Books.

Satterly, Faye. 2004. *Where Have All the Nurses Gone? The Impact of the Nursing Shortage of American Healthcare.* Amherst, NY: Prometheus Books.

Savage, Jan. 1987. *Nurses, Gender, and Sexuality.* London: Heinemann Nursing.

———. 1995. *Nursing Intimacy: An Ethnographic Approach to Nurse-Patient Interaction.* London: Scutari Press.

Scherzer, Teresa. 2003. "The Race and Class of Women's Work." *Race, Gender, and Class* 10:23–42.

Schwalbe, Michael, and Michelle Wolkomir. 2001. "The Masculine Self as Problem and Resource in Interview Studies of Men." *Men and Masculinities* 4:90–103.

Shapiro, Michael M. 1998. "A Career Ladder Based on Benner's Model: An Analysis of Expected Outcomes." *Journal of Nursing Administration* 28:13–19.

Shattell, Mona. 2004. "Nurse-Patient Interaction: A Review of the Literature." *Journal of Clinical Nursing* 13:714–722.

Smith, Barbara. 1983. *Home Girls: A Black Feminist Anthology.* Latham, NY: Kitchen Table Women of Color Press.

Smith, Dorothy. 1987. *The Everyday World as Problematic: A Feminist Sociology.* Boston: Northeastern University Press.

———. 1990. *The Conceptual Practices of Power: A Feminist Sociology of Knowledge.* Boston: Northeastern University Press.

———. 1997. "Comment on Hekman's 'Truth and Method: Feminist Standpoint Theory Revisited.'" *Signs* 22:392–398.

———. 2005. *Institutional Ethnography: A Sociology for People.* Lanham, MD: Alta Mira Press.

Spelman, Elizabeth. 1988. *Inessential Woman.* Boston: Beacon Press.

Stacey, Judith. 1988. "Can There Be a Feminist Ethnography?" *Women's Studies International Forum* 2:21–27.

Strauss, Anselm L., and Juliet Corbin. 1990. *Basics of Qualitative Research: Grounded Theory Procedures and Techniques.* Newbury Park, CA: Sage.

Swanson Kristen. M. 1991. "Empirical Development of a Middle Range Theory of Caring." *Nursing Research* 40:161–166.

Takahashi, Aya. 2004. *The Development of the Japanese Nursing Profession: Adopting and Adapting Western Influences.* New York: RoutledgeTwine, France Winddance. 2000. "Racial Ideologies and Racial Methodologies." In *Racing Research, Researching Race: Methodological Dilemmas in Critical Race Studies,* edited by France Winddance Twine and Jonathan W. Warren, 1–34. New York: New York University Press.

Warren, Jonathan W. 2000. "Masters in the Field: White Talk, White Privilege, White Biases." In *Racing Research, Researching Race: Methodological Dilemmas in Critical Race Studies,* edited by France Winddance Twine and Jonathan W. Warren, 135–164. New York: New York University Press.

Watson, Jean 2003. "Love and Caring: Ethics of Face and Hand." *Nursing Administration Quarterly* 27:197–202.

———. 2005. *Caring Science as Sacred Science.* Philadelphia: F.A. Davis.

Weinburg, Dana Beth. 2003. *Code Green: Money-Driven Hospitals and the Dismantling of Nursing.* Ithaca, NY: Cornell University Press.

Weiss, Robert. 1994. *Learning from Strangers: The Art and Method of Qualitative Interview Studies.* New York: Maxwell Macmillan International.

Welsh, Sandy, Jacquie Carr, Barbara Macquarrie, and Audrey Huntley. 2006. "'I'm Not Thinking of It as Sexual Harassment': Understanding Harassment across Race and Citizenship." *Gender and Society* 20:87–107.

Welter, Barbara. 1966. "The Cult of True Womanhood, 1820–1860." *American Quarterly* 18:151–174.

West, Candace, and Don Zimmerman. 1987. "Doing Gender." *Gender and Society* 1 (2): 125–151.

Whittock, Margaret, and Laurence Leonard. 2003. "Stepping outside the Stereotype: A Pilot Study of the Motivations and Experiences of Males in the Nursing Professions." *Journal of Nursing Management* 11:242–249.

Williams, Angela. 2001a. "A Literature on the Concept of Intimacy in Nursing." *Journal of Advanced Nursing* 33:660–667.

———. 2001b. "A Study of Practising Nurses' Perceptions and Experiences of Intimacy within the Nurse-Patient Relationship." *Journal of Advanced Nursing* 35 (2): 188–196.

Williams, Christine L. 1993. *Doing "Women's Work."* Thousand Oaks, CA: Sage.

———. 1995. *Still a Man's World: Men Who Do Women's Work.* Berkeley: University of California Press.

Wolf, Zane Robinson. 1988. *Nurses' Work: The Sacred and the Profane.* Philadelphia: University of Pennsylvania Press.

Woodward, Vivien M. 1997. "Professional Caring: A Contradiction in Terms?" *Journal of Advanced Nursing* 26:999–1004.

Zelizer, Viviana A. 2005. *The Purchase of Intimacy.* Princeton, NJ: Princeton University Press.

————. 2009. "Intimacy in Economic Organizations." In *Economic Sociology of Work*, edited by Nina Bandelj, 23–55. Bingley, UK: Emerald.

————. 2010. "Caring Everywhere." In *Intimate Labors: Cultures, Technologies, and the Politics of Care*, edited by Eileen Boris and Rhacel Salazar Perrenas, 267–279. Palo Alto, CA: Stanford University Press.

Zerubavel, Eviatar. 2006. *The Elephant in the Room: Silence and Denial in Everyday Life*, Oxford: Oxford University Press.

Zinn, Maxine Baca. 1979. "Field Research in Minority Communities: Ethical, Methodological, and Political Observations by an Insider." *Social Problems* 27:209–219.

Zinn, Maxine Baca, Lynn Weber Cannon, Elizabeth Higginbotham, and Bonnie Thornton Dill. 1990. "The Costs of Exclusionary Practices in Women's Studies" In *Making Face, Making Soul: Creative and Critical Perspectives by Women of Color*, edited by Gloria Anzaldua, 29–41. San Francisco: Aunt Lute Foundation.

Index

Lisa C. Ruchti is an Assistant Professor in the Women's and Gender Studies program and the Department of Anthropology and Sociology at West Chester University of Pennsylvania. Her research and teaching focus on the sociology of gender, intersectionality, and transnational feminist theories.